KETO DIETS

3 books set

The only guideline for keto diets you will ever need

Keto Diet For Begginers

14-Day Ketogenic Diet Weight Loss Plan
with 28 Easy Low-Carb Recipes.

By:

Holly R.Evans

TABLE OF CONTENTS

INTRODUCTION

Anxious to lose some weight and looking for something that can burn fat at maximum speed? Have you tried endless other diet plans but nothing seems to work for more than a few weeks? For many people, the ketogenic diet is a great option for weight loss. It is very different and allows the person on the diet to eat a diet that consists of foods that you may not expect.

So the ketogenic diet, or keto, is a diet that consists of very low carbs and high fat. How many diets are there where you can start your day off with bacon and eggs, loads of it, then follow it up with chicken wings for lunch and then steak and broccoli for dinner. That may sound too good to be true for many. Well on this diet this is a great day of eating and you followed the rules perfectly with that meal plan.

When you eat a very low amount of carbs your body gets put into a state of ketosis. What this means is your body burns fat for energy. How low of an amount of carbs do you need to eat in order to get into ketosis? Well, it varies from person to person, but it is a safe bet to stay under 25 net carbs. Many would suggest that when you are in the "induction phase" which is when you are actually putting your body into ketosis, you should stay under 10 net carbs.

If you aren't sure what net carbs are, let me help you. Net carbs are the amount of carbs you eat minus the amount of dietary fiber. So if on the day you eat a total of 35 grams of net carbs and 13 grams of dietary fiber, your net carbs for the day would be 22.

WHAT IS THE KETO DIET?

The Keto diet involves going long spells on extremely low (no higher than 30g per day) to almost zero g per day of carbs and increasing your fats to a really high level (to the point where they may make up as much as 65% of your daily macronutrients intake.) The idea behind this is to get your body into a state of ketosis. In this state of ketosis the body is supposed to be more inclined to use fat for energy- and research says it does just this. Depleting your carbohydrate/glycogen liver stores and then moving onto fat for fuel means you should end up being shredded.

HOW DOES IT WORK?

The keto diet aims to force your body into using a different type of fuel. Instead of relying on sugar (glucose) that comes from carbohydrates (such as grains, legumes, vegetables, and fruits), the keto diet relies on ketone bodies, a type of fuel that the liver produces from stored fat.

Burning fat seems like an ideal way to lose pounds. But getting the liver to make ketone bodies is tricky:

- It requires that you deprive yourself of carbohydrates, fewer than 20 to 50 grams of carbs per day (keep in mind that a medium-sized banana has about 27 grams of carbs).

- It typically takes a few days to reach a state of ketosis.

- Eating too much protein can interfere with ketosis.

WHAT DO YOU EAT?

Because the keto diet has such a high fat requirement, followers must eat fat at each meal. In a daily 2,000-calorie diet, that might look like 165 grams of fat, 40 grams of carbs, and 75 grams of protein. However, the exact ratio depends on your particular needs.

Some healthy unsaturated fats are allowed on the keto diet — like nuts (almonds, walnuts), seeds, avocados, tofu, and olive oil. But saturated fats from oils (palm, coconut), lard, butter, and cocoa butter are encouraged in high amounts.

Protein is part of the keto diet, but it doesn't typically discriminate between lean protein foods and protein sources high in saturated fat such as beef, pork, and bacon.

What about fruits and vegetables? All fruits are rich in carbs, but you can have certain fruits (usually berries) in small portions. Vegetables (also rich in carbs) are restricted to leafy greens (such as kale, Swiss chard, spinach), cauliflower, broccoli, Brussels sprouts, asparagus, bell peppers, onions, garlic, mushrooms, cucumber, celery, and summer squashes. A cup of chopped broccoli has about six carbs.

KETO RISKS

A ketogenic diet has numerous risks. Top of the list: it's high in saturated fat. McManus recommends that you keep saturated fats to no more than 7% of your daily calories because of the link to heart disease. And indeed, the keto diet is associated with an increase in "bad" LDL cholesterol, which is also linked to heart disease.

Other potential keto risks include these:

Diarrhea

If you find yourself running to the bathroom more often while on a ketogenic diet, a quick internet search will show you that you're not alone. (Yes, people are tweeting about keto diarrhea.) This may be due to the gallbladder—the organ that produces bile to help break down fat in the diet—feeling "overwhelmed," says Axe.

Diarrhea can also be due to a lack of fiber in the diet, says Kizer, which can happen when someone cuts way back on carbs (like whole-grain bread and pasta) and doesn't supplement with other fiber-rich foods, like vegetables. It can also be caused by an intolerance to dairy or artificial sweeteners—

things you might be eating more of since switching to a high-fat, low-carb lifestyle.

Nutrient deficiency.

"If you're not eating a wide variety of vegetables, fruits, and grains, you may be at risk for deficiencies in micronutrients, including selenium, magnesium, phosphorus, and vitamins B and C," says registered dietitian Kathy McManus, director of the Department of Nutrition at Harvard-affiliated Brigham and Women's Hospital.

Liver problems. With so much fat to metabolize, the diet could make any existing liver conditions worse.

Kidney problems.

The kidneys help metabolize protein, and McManus says the keto diet may overload them. (The current recommended intake for protein averages 46 grams per day for women, and 56 grams for men).

Less Muscle Mass, Decreased Metabolism

Another consequence of keto-related weight changes can be a loss of muscle mass, says Kristen Kizer, RD, a nutritionist at Houston Methodist

Medical Center.—especially if you're eating much more fat than protein. "You'll lose weight, but it might actually be a lot of muscle," she says, "and because muscle burns more calories than fat, that will affect your metabolism."

When a person goes off the ketogenic diet and regains much of their original weight, it's often not in the same proportions, says Kizer: Instead of regaining lean muscle, you're likely to regain fat. "Now you're back to your starting weight, but you no longer have the muscle mass to burn the calories that you did before," she says. "That can have lasting effects on your resting metabolic rate, and on your weight long-term."

Constipation

The keto diet is low in fibrous foods like grains and legumes.

Fuzzy thinking and mood swings

"The brain needs sugar from healthy carbohydrates to function. Low-carb diets may cause confusion and irritability," says McManus.

HOW TO LOSE OVER 25LBS IN 8 WEEKS WITHOUT HARMFUL EXERCISES AND TO SAVE OVER 100$/WEEK

Although exercise can certainly help build fat-burning muscle and maintain a svelte physi?ue, it won't shrink your waistline as much as changing your diet will. So now that we know "eating less" should take priority in your weight-loss journey, where to start? Because it's easier said than done, we've uncovered slimming secrets that can help you tackle your muffin top through diet swaps as well as lifestyle and eating habit changes.

Check this out how you can avoid becoming a gym rat below, and then double down on your efforts by with healthy recipes, supermarket shopping guides, and essential nutrition tips delivered to your doorstep.

Refrain from Alcohol

Cut down your alcohol and sugar consumption, and limit saturated and trans fats, as these can wreak havoc on your weight-loss efforts and your health. Avoid sugar from desserts, fruits in syrup, and soda. Steer clear of unhealthy fats, which are present in baked and fried foods, hard margarine, lard, fatty meats and full-fat dairy products. Choose healthy fats from olive or canola oil and soft margarine instead.

Eat Healthy Fats

When you're trying to lose weight, the last thing you want to do is eat anything fatty, right? Wrong. You just have to make sure you're eating the right kind of fat. While eating certain types of fat are definitely no-nos when you're trying to lose weight — looking at you, saturated fat! — adding healthy fats into your diet is a game-changer. Research has shown eating good-for-you fats like avocado on a daily basis — even if that's just throwing some onto your salad for lunch — can leave you so full and satisfied that you're not reaching for unhealthy, sugary snacks later on. And without all those excess calories, you're bound to drop unwanted weight.

Hop on the Yoga Bandwagon

You might not see yoga as a solid weight-loss method, but think again. Aside from working out every muscle in your body and reducing your stress levels, you're also raising your heart rate to reap some major fat-burning benefits. Try this workout that's designed to help you drop pounds and tone up in process.

Dance the Weight Off

The best types of workouts are the ones you're having so much fun during that you forget you're even working out in the first place. If you want to lose weight, try this 35-minute by Body by Simone creator Simone de la Rue. You'll be sweating in no time.

Increase Your H20 Intake

Here's your permission to dump that electric-green juice craze down the drain. A better plan is to sip water throughout the day. Research shows it actually helps you cut down on calories. Often, thirst is confused for hunger. And try salt water, while you're at it. When it comes to H20, salt is not the enemy. "Water needs electrolytes like sodium, potassium, and chloride to be best absorbed," says Jenny Westerkamp, an R.D. in Chicago, which explains why they're added to popular sports drinks.

She recommends adding a pinch of Celtic sea salt or real salt (unrefined and unbleached) to your water before chugging. "The electrolytes in the salt will push water into the cells where they need to be, rather than letting the water get flushed out, causing you to go to the bathroom every other minute." You'll notice a spike in energy after staying hydrated, too, and you'll be less likely to give in to cravings which are even harder to avoid when you're running on empty.

Rethink What "Exercise" Really Means

We know we said these tips were about shedding pounds without working out, but being active is important, so here's radical idea: Change the way you think about exercise by choosing to do something you enjoy. "It doesn't have to be in a gym," Christy Harrison, a Brooklyn-based dietitian, says. "It could be a dance class or going for a run around your neighborhood." And it might even be worth it to get into tree pose when you've only got a few minutes. A study published in the journal PLOS ONE found that just 10 minutes of exercise has huge health benefits.

Give Meal-Prepping a Try

Yeah, yeah — meal-prepping isn't exciting. That's nothing new. But by spending a few hours every weekend preparing some meals for the week ahead, you could see a lot of progress in a short amount of time. Plus, you'll save money by cutting back on the delivery. "When you plan an entire week of dinner in advance, you're way less likely to go off course and indulge in foods that aren't good for you," says Pamela Salzman, a certified holistic health expert and cooking instructor. Start with making your lunches in advance and go from there.

Get Smart About Nutrition

Crying tears of sugar because you ate a donut that isn't on your approved list of foods isn't going to do you any good. You ate a donut. Cool. Move on. Here's why: Remember when you were a kid and your mom banned soda from your life forever and it only led to serious root beer binges when you got to your friend's house? Those same rules are in play here. Get label-crazed and you'll lose your mind — not excess weight. And cutting yourself off from all of your favorite things will only lead to overdoing it on the sugary, salty foods.

Instead, Harrison, says. you should look at foods as a way of self-care — eat what makes you feel good and forget about it as a means of slimming down (although a solid side effect of healthy eating: weight loss). Does that mean a free-for-all on the candy bowl? No. But it's a rule your body will naturally adapt to, not something you have to force on it. A bowl of almonds made you feel amazing in the mid-afternoon sales meeting, but those red gummies, not so much. Next time, you'll likely reach for the almonds.

BEST KETO-FRIENDLY DRINKS

If you're on a ketogenic diet, you're super focused on what you're eating and especially what you're not eating. But don't forget that what you sip can set you up for success, too.

Bear in mind, that going Keto means you can't have alcohol, right? Here's a list of Keto Friendly drinks

Water Is the Best Drink You Can Sip on the Keto Diet

This is hands down the best drink for you — keto or not, says Keene. Keep a water bottle near you at all times and sip throughout the day to stay ahead of your hydration.

Tea

Tea is another great option for keto, and if you don't add anything to it, it's perfectly keto-friendly, too. There are a lot of different tea varieties, and if you're new to tea, we recommend experimenting with a few types to find out what you like the most.

Black Tea

This is the strongest, and usually has the highest caffeine content. Similarly to coffee, there are a lot of different kinds of black teas out there – there are lots of different sorts of tea, from different countries of origin (Indian black tea, such as Assam and Darjeeling being one of the most popular ones, for example), with different flavours, and so on.

Green Tea

This is also extremely popular and readily available in almost any supermarket or health food store around the world.

Seltzer or Sparkling Water Is Another Carb-Free Drink Option

This is a great way to mix up your usual water — just avoid tonic, which looks like clear, plain bubbled water, but actually contains a ton of sugar. Adding a squeeze of lemon adds nearly ½ gram (g) of carbohydrates, notes the U.S. Department of Agriculture (USDA).

Plain Coffee, or Coffee With Unsweetened Heavy Cream, Is Also Okay on the Keto Diet

Like with tea, it's what you add to your brew that matters most. Drinking it black is completely calorie free, but many keto dieters will appreciate the added fat that heavy cream provides, says Scott Keatley, RDN, of Keatley Medical Nutrition Therapy in New York City. For adults, up to 400 milligrams (mg) per day of caffeine is considered safe, according to the Mayo Clinic. For reference, 1 cup — 8 fluid ounces (oz) — of coffee contains about 92 mg, per the USDA, while a tall coffee at Starbucks contains 245 mg, according to the company website.

Diet Soda

Like soda, but without the sugar and the calories.

Juice Alternatives

There are also some low-calorie and zero calorie drinks like Powerade Zero and Vitamin Water Zero that taste good and hydrate you without the extra sugar. Just make sure you read the labels of any tasty low-calorie drink you buy because they may have added sugars.

Low-Carb Dairy Products and Dairy Alternatives

A little bit of milk in your coffee or tea is okay, but don't have too much. If you need to use more than a couple of tablespoons of milk, try using heavy cream or a dairy alternative like unsweetened coconut milk or almond milk instead.

Energy Drinks

Most energy drinks are packed with more sugar than soda, but there are many low-carb and zero carb energy drinks on the market. However, just because it says "low-carb" on the container doesn't mean that it will fit within your daily carb limit. Always read labels carefully, especially when you are purchasing energy drinks.

Bone Broth Can Be a Comforting Keto-Friendly Drink

There's something uniquely warming and comforting about sipping a steaming cup of bone broth. One brand notes this liquid offers 0 carbs and 1 cup contains less than 50 calories while adding 9 g of protein. Traditional broth is a stellar option, too, though it has less protein. One cup contains 13 calories and 2.5 g of protein, according to the USDA.

Nut Milks Are Also Low-Carb and Okay for Keto Dieters

Almond, coconut, and cashew milks make for great choices if you want to mix things up, as they contain 1 g (or less) of carbs per cup. Just be sure to always read the nutrition label closely and choose unsweetened varieties. These are often fortified with vitamins and minerals, so they're a good way to get in calcium and vitamin D.

THE 7 IMPORTANT THINGS YOU SHOULD KNOW ABOUT THE KETO DIET BEFORE YOU START

The keto diet has go vira in popularity, and it's because going keto has helped celebrites like Gwyneth Paltrow, Halle Berry, Kim Kardashian used Keto to transform their bodies and many people to lose their weight, in some cases more than 150 pounds. But the diet, which is high in fat, is also controversial, as dietitians worry about the implications of cutting out an entire food group (grains and carbs) and eating an abundance of saturated fat.

But if you're curious about embarking on the keto diet, here's everything you need to know before getting started.

Keto is more than a diet.

It's a way of eating (WOE). You'll often hear people describe their keto diet as a "lifestyle" or "way of eating." That's because it's not something you can stop and start like most other diets. In fact, going on and off keto can mess up your metabolism and confuse your body, possibly causing you to gain more weight. For keto to be effective in enhancing your health, helping you lose weight, and improving your mental focus and energy levels, you must be consistent and make it a permanent lifestyle change.

Keto requires time.

You'll hear about keto success stories where weight starts to melt off almost immediately. Those cases are typically associated with people who have lots of weight to lose. In general, the more weight you have to lose, the faster it'll come off at the beginning. Another thing to keep in mind is that slow and steady weight loss is healthier, more sustainable, and more likely to stay off. So be patient with yourself. Don't give up on the keto diet because you don't immediately see drastic weight loss.

Keto can be customized.

The ketogenic diet – generally speaking – is 75% fat, 20% protein, 5% carbohydrates. But daily carb intake can vary from 20 grams to 50 grams depending on how your body processes carbs. There's no magic number of carbs that'll get you into ketosis. If you're not losing weight or unable to get into ketosis at 50 grams, keep dropping your carb macros until you achieve the results you want. Bottom line: do what works for you.

Going keto can impact your workouts.

You may lose some strength and endurance at the beginning of your keto diet. This is because your body is used to burning carbs for fuel, and it suddenly doesn't have that option anymore. As it adjusts to burning fat, you'll notice that your workout capacity will return to normal. And you may even notice that your athletic performance improves once your body is fully keto-adapted and burning fat for fuel.

Stick With It

After that initial shedding period, the weight loss may slow significantly. But that's ok. As your body gets used to the diet you'll likely lose weight over time—which is actually healthier and more sustainable than losing a lot of weight overnight.

Stay Hydrated

Since you lose a lot of water weight on Keto, especially at first, it's crucial to drink a lot of water to stay hydrated. Drink more than you are used to as you are changing the way your body is functioning. Increase your salt intake as well to help retain water and prevent dehydration (a common side effect of the diet).

The biggest mistake people make while on Keto, you can avoid this

Eating Too Much Protein

To some of you, this may not seem like such a bad thing. You aren't allowed many carbs so a way to supplement that is through consuming protein.

However, having too much protein is going to have negative effects on your body during a keto diet.

Your body only needs so much protein, anything more than that and it starts to get converted into fat. We are trying to eliminate fat so anything that adds fat to your body is a negative.

Avoiding this is pretty simple. All you need to do is focus on your macros. Stay with your macros and you won't have to worry about having anything in excess. You will only have exactly what you need.

KETO DIETING? HERE ARE 10 FOODS YOU MUST HAVE IN YOUR KITCHEN

Because we are surrounded by fast food restaurants and processed meals, it can be a challenge to avoid carb-rich foods, but proper planning can help.

Plan menus and snacks at least a week ahead of time, so you aren't caught with only high carb meal choices. Research keto recipes online; there are quite a few good ones to choose from. Immerse yourself in the keto lifestyle, find your favorite recipes, and stick with them.

There are a few items that are staples of a keto diet. Be sure to have these items on hand:

- **Eggs** - Used in omelets, quiches (yes, heavy cream is legal on keto!), hard boiled as a snack, low carb pizza crust, and more; if you like eggs, you have a great chance of success on this diet
- **Bacon** - Do I need a reason? breakfast, salad garnish, burger topper, BLT's (no bread of course; try a BLT in a bowl, tossed in mayo)

- **Cream cheese** - Dozens of recipes, pizza crusts, main dishes, desserts
- **Shredded cheese** - Sprinkle over taco meat in a bowl, made into tortilla chips in the microwave, salad toppers, low-carb pizza and enchiladas
- **Lots of romaine and spinach** - Fill up on the green veggies; have plenty on hand for a quick salad when hunger pangs hit
- **EZ-Sweetz liquid sweetener -** Use a couple of drops in place of sugar; this artificial sweetener is the most natural and easiest to use that I've found
- **Cauliflower** - Fresh or frozen bags you can eat this low-carb veggie by itself, tossed in olive oil and baked, mashed in fake potatoes, chopped/shredded and used in place of rice under main dishes, in low-carb and keto pizza crusts, and much more
- **Frozen chicken tenders** - Have a large bag on hand; thaw quickly and grill, saute, mix with veggies and top with garlic sauce in a low carb flatbread, use in Chicken piccata, chicken alfredo, tacos, enchiladas, Indian Butter chicken, and more
- **Ground beef** - Make a big burger and top with all sorts of things from cheese, to sauteed mushrooms, to grilled onions... or

crumble and cook with taco seasoning and use in provolone cheese taco shells; throw in a dish with lettuce, avocado, cheese, sour cream for a tortilla-less taco salad

- **Almonds (plain or flavored)** - these are a tasty and healthy snack; however, be sure to count them as you eat, because the carbs DO add up. Flavors include habanero, coconut, salt and vinegar and more.

28 CHEEP, TASTY KETO FRIENDLY RECIPIES

The Ketogenic diet trend has already given us some amazing new ways to enjoy our food and we aren't going to lie, we are loving every minute of it! Is the Keto diet right for you?

Here are Keto Friendly recipies you can try in the kitchen or order in your favourite restaurants. You can still out to eat with your friends.

BreakFast

Keto Chicken Parmesan

"A delicious keto-friendly chicken Parmesan. Enjoy a classic Italian dish, and keep your macros in check!"

Ingredients

2 servings
442 cals
Prep: 20 m
Cook: 8 m
Total: 28

- 1 (8 ounce) skinless, boneless chicken breast
- 1 egg
- 1 tablespoon heavy whipping cream
- 1 1/2 ounces pork rinds, crushed
- 1 ounce grated Parmesan cheese
- 1/2 teaspoon salt
- 1/2 teaspoon garlic powder
- 1/2 teaspoon red pepper flakes (optional)
- 1/2 teaspoon ground black pepper

- 1/2 teaspoon Italian seasoning
- 1/2 cup jarred tomato sauce (such as Rao's®)
- 1/4 cup shredded mozzarella cheese
- 1 tablespoon ghee (clarified butter)
- Add all ingredients to list

Instructions

- Set oven rack about 6 inches from the heat source and preheat the oven's broiler.
- Slice chicken breast through the middle horizontally from one side to within 1/2 inch of the other side. Open the two sides and spread them out like an open book. Pound chicken flat until about 1/2-inch thick.
- Beat egg and cream together in a bowl.
- Combine crushed pork rinds, Parmesan cheese, salt, garlic powder, red pepper flakes, ground black pepper, and Italian seasoning in bowl; transfer breading to a plate.
- Dip chicken into egg mixture; coat completcly. Press chicken into breading; thickly coat both sides.
- Heat a skillet over medium-high heat; add ghee. Place chicken in the pan; cook until no

longer pink in the center and the juices run clear, about 3 minutes per side. An instant-read thermometer inserted into the center should read at least 165 degrees F (74 degrees C). Be careful to keep breading in place.

- Transfer chicken to a baking sheet. Cover with tomato sauce; top with mozzarella cheese.
- Broil until cheese is bubbling and barely browned, about 2 minutes.

Nutrition

Serving Size: 1 Calories: 509 Fat: 28g Carbohydrates: 10.5g Fiber: 6g

Keto mushroom omelet

Looking for a ⬚uick and easy way to start your day? This hearty omelet is super healthy, and just takes a few minutes to make! Fresh mushrooms make a delicious filling. Enjoy this keto meal anytime

Time: 5 + 10 m
kcal: 510

Ingredients

- 3 eggs
- 1 oz. butter, for frying
- 1 oz. shredded cheese
- 1/5 yellow onion
- 3 mushrooms
- salt and pepper

Instructions

- Crack the eggs into a mixing bowl with a pinch of salt and pepper. Whisk the eggs with a fork until smooth and frothy.
- Add salt and spices to taste.
- Melt butter in a frying pan. Once the butter has melted, pour in the egg mixture.

- When the omelet begins to cook and get firm, but still has a little raw egg on top, sprinkle cheese, mushrooms and onion on top (optional).
- Using a spatula, carefully ease around the edges of the omelet, and then fold it over in half. When it starts to turn golden brown underneath, remove the pan from the heat and slide the omelet on to a plate.

Recipe Note!

Serve the omelet with a crispy, green salad with vinaigrette dressing on the side. Yum!

Nutrition Info
Net carbs: 3 % (4 g)
Fiber: 1 g
Fat: 77 % (43 g)
Protein: 20 % (25 g)
kcal: 510

Keto Pancakes

There's nothing like a big stack of pancakes for breakfast—they're a breakfast staple! Just because you're on the Keto diet doesn't mean you've gotta miss out on the joys of flapjacks. This recipe is super easy and will definitely satisfy your craving.

Yields: 10
Prep Time: 0 hours 5 mins
Total Time: 0 hours 15 mins

Ingredients

- 1/2 c. almond flour
- 4 oz. cream cheese, softened
- 4 large eggs
- 1 tsp. lemon zest
- Butter, for frying and serving

Instructions

- In a medium bowl, whisk together almond flour, cream cheese, eggs, and lemon zest until smooth.

- In a nonstick skillet over medium heat, melt 1 tablespoon butter. Pour in about 3 tablespoons batter and cook until golden, 2 minutes. Flip and cook 2 minutes more. Transfer to a plate and continue with the rest of the batter.
- Serve topped with butter.

Recipe Note
Total recipe yields 4-6 small pancakes.

Nutrition Facts
Calories 339 Calories from Fat 270
Potassium 145mg 4%
Total Carbohydrates 7g 2%
Dietary Fiber 3g 12%
Sugars 1g
Protein 12g 24

Keto Banana Nut Muffins

Tired of eggs for keto breakfast? These Keto Banana Nut Muffins are so simple and delicious, your kids will love helping you make them on the weekends just as much as they'll love helping you eat them!

Prep Time: 10 Minutes
Cook Time: 20 Minutes
Total Time: 30 minutes
Yield: 10 Muffins

Ingredients

Muffin Battter

- 1 1/4 Cup almond flour (I use this)
- 1/2 Cup powdered erythritol (I use this)
- 2 tablespoons ground flax (feel free to omit if you don't have it...it just adds a bit more depth to the flavors)
- 2 teaspoons baking powder
- 1/2 teaspoons ground cinnamon
- 5 tablespoon butter, melted
- 2 1/2 teaspoons banana extract
- 1 teaspoon vanilla extract
- 1/4 cup unsweetened almond milk

- 1/4 cup sour cream
- 2 eggs

Walnut Crumble

- 3/4 cup chopped walnuts
- 1 tablespoon butter, cold and cut in 4 pieces
- 1 tablespoon almond flour
- 1 tablespoon powdered erythritol

Instructions

- Preheat oven to 350

- Prepare muffin tin with 10 paper liners, and set aside

- In a large bowl, mix almond flour, erythritol (or preferred sweetener) flax, baking powder and cinnamon

- Stir in butter, banana extract, vanilla extract, almond milk, and sour cream.

- Add eggs to mixture and gently stir until fully combined.

- Fill muffin tins about 1/2-3/4 full with mixture.

- **If you need more accurate measurements, weigh the batter on a food scale and divide by 10. That will give you the grams of batter per cup.

Crumble Topping

- Add walnuts, butter, and almond flour to food processor.

- Pulse a few times until nuts are chopped into small pieces. If mixture seems too dry (sometimes some walnuts are softer than others) feel free to add another tablespoon of butter.

- Sprinkle bits of the mixture evenly over batter and gently press down.

- Sprinkle erythritol on top of crumble mixture.

- Bake for 20 minutes or until golden and toothpick comes out clean. Let cool for at least 30 minutes, an hour or more if possible. This lets them firm up.

- *If they seem to be cooking faster, take them out sooner to avoid burning. Alternatively, if they are still wet looking, return them to the oven for a few minutes keeping a close eye on them.

Nutrition Info
Calories: 184
Total Carbs: 7g
Fiber: 3g
Net Carbs: 4g
Protein: 7g
Fat: 14g

Keto Fat Bombs

These fat bombs are your best friend. Don't let the name scare you—these little balls are the perfect way to curb your hunger.

Yields: 8
Prep Time: 0 hours 5 mins
Total Time: 0 hours 25 mins

Ingredients

- 8 oz. cream cheese, softened to room temperature
- 1/2 c. keto-friendly peanut butter
- 1/4 c. coconut oil, plus 2 tbsp.
- 1/2 tsp. kosher salt
- 1 c. keto-friendly dark chocolate chips (such as Lily's)

Instructions

- Line a small baking sheet with parchment paper. In a medium bowl, combine cream cheese, peanut butter, ¼ c coconut oil, and salt. Using a hand mixer, beat mixture until fully combined, about 2 minutes. Place bowl in freezer to firm up slightly, 10 to 15 minutes.

- When peanut butter mixture has hardened, use a small cookie scoop or spoon to create golf ball sized balls. Place in the refrigerator to harden, 5 minutes.
- Meanwhile, make chocolate drizzle: combine chocolate chips and remaining coconut oil in a microwave safe bowl and microwave in 30 second intervals until fully melted. Drizzle over peanut butter balls and place back in the refrigerator to harden, 5 minutes. Serve.
- To store, keep covered in refrigerator.

Nutrition Info

Per Serving: 84 calories; 8.4 g fat; 2.6 g carbohydrates; 2 g protein; 0 mg cholesterol; 0 mg sodium

Zucchini Egg Cups

Yields: 12
Prep Time: 0 hours 10 mins
Total Time: 0 hours 40 mins

Ingredients

- Cooking spray, for pan
- 2 zucchini, peeled into strips
- 1/4 lb. ham, chopped
- 1/2 c. cherry tomatoes, quartered
- 8 eggs
- 1/2 c. heavy cream
- Kosher salt
- Freshly ground black pepper
- 1/2 tsp. dried oregano
- 1 c. Pinch red pepper flakes
- 1 c. shredded cheddar

Instructions

- Preheat oven to 400° and grease a muffin tin with cooking spray. Line the inside and bottom of the muffin tin with zucchini strips, to form a crust. Sprinkle ham and cherry tomatoes inside each crust.

- In a medium bowl whisk together eggs, heavy, cream, oregano, and red pepper flakes then season with salt and pepper. Pour egg mixture over ham and tomatoes then top with cheese.
- Bake until eggs are set, 30 minutes.

Ham & Cheese Breakfast Roll-Ups

Yields: 2
Prep Time: 0 hours 20 mins
Total Time: 0 hours 20 mins

Ingredients

- 4 large eggs
- 1/4 c. milk
- 2 tbsp. Chopped chives
- kosher salt
- Freshly ground black pepper
- 1 tbsp. butter
- 1 c. shredded cheddar, divided
- 4 slices ham

Instructions

- In a medium bowl, whisk together eggs, milk, and chives. Season with salt and pepper.
- In a medium skillet over medium heat, melt butter. Pour half of the egg mixture into the skillet, moving to create a thin layer that covers the entire pan.
- Cook for 2 minutes. Add 1/2 cup cheddar and cover for 2 minutes more, until the

cheese is melty. Remove onto plate, place 2 slices of ham, and roll tightly. Repeat with remaining ingredients and serve.

Nutrition Info

Calories: 260
Fat: 21 g
Saturated Fat: 11 g
Trans Fat: 0.5 g
Sodium: 530 mg
Sugars: 1 g
Protein: 17 g
Fibre: 0 g
Carbohydrate: 0 g

Curry Tofu Scramble with Avocado

This tofu scramble is a fabulous low carb veggie lover approach to begin the morning, with a lot of supplements and sufficient calories togive you vitality for the day ahead.

Prep Time 5 minutes;
Cook Time 13 minutes;
Total Time 20 minutes,
Calories 380 kcal
Servings 3

Ingredients:

- 1 tbsp coconut oil
- 2 tbsp olive oil
- 300 g tofu (extra firm)
- 1 tsp turmeric
- 1 tbsp nutritional yeast
- 1 tbsp curry powder
- 1/2 cup zucchini (chopped)
- 1 cup mushrooms (chopped)
- 1 tomato (chopped)
- cilantro (optional)(to garnish)
- 300-gram avocado

Instructions

- The initial step is to dry the tofu so it ingests the flavor.
- Cut the tofu into 1 inch long strips, spread out the strips on a paper towel,
- put another paper towel to finish everything and after that a slashing board.
- Place something substantial over this, for example, a few books.
- Abandon it to sit for around 15 minutes.
- Add the coconut oil to the dish and disintegrate the tofu into the skillet with your hands.
- Cook for around 5 minutes, mixing every now and again.
- Include the turmeric, nourishing yeast and curry powder and 1 tbsp of the olive oil,
- blend and cook for a further 4 minutes.
- Add whatever remains of the olive oil, zucchini, mushroom and tomato and sear for a further 4 minutes blending much of the time.
- Serve with 1 little medium size avocado (roughly 100g) cut.

Recipe Notes:
This meal can be refrigerated for a few days.
Nutritional Information:
Calories: 381, Fats: 32g, Protein: 11g, Net Carbs: 8g

Avocado Egg Boats

Prep Time: 0 hours 10 mins
Total Time: 0 hours 30 mins

Ingredients

- 2 ripe avocados, pitted and halved
- 4 large eggs
- kosher salt
- Freshly ground black pepper
- 3 slices bacon
- Freshly chopped chives, for garnish

Instructions

- Preheat oven to 350°. Place avocados in a baking dish, then crack eggs into a bowl. Using a spoon, transfer yolks to each avocado half, then spoon in as much egg white as you can fit without spilling over.
- Season with salt and pepper and bake until whites are set and yolks are no longer runny, about 20 minutes. (Cover with foil if avocados are beginning to brown.)
- Meanwhile, in a large skillet over medium heat, cook bacon until crisp, 8 minutes, then

transfer to a paper towel-lined plate and chop.
- Top avocados with bacon and chives and serve with a spoon.

Nutrition Info
Calories 251

Keto Cannoli Stuffed Crepes

These Keto Cannoli Stuffed Crepes are perfect for any special occasion breakfast or brunch! Tastes like you're cheating, but they are low carb, gluten free, grain free, Atkins, and nut free too!

Prep Time: 15 minutes
Cook Time: 20 minutes
Total Time: 35 minutes
Yield: 4 servings

Ingredients

For the crepes:

- 8 ounces cream cheese, softened
- 8 eggs
- 1/2 teaspoon ground cinnamon
- 1 tablespoon granulated erythritol sweetener
- 2 tablespoons butter, for the pan

For the cannoli filling:

- 6 ounces mascarpone cheese, softened
- 1 cup whole milk ricotta cheese
- 1/2 teaspoon lemon zest

- 1/2 teaspoon ground cinnamon
- 1/4 teaspoon unsweetened vanilla extract
- 1/4 cup powdered erythritol sweetener

For the optional chocolate drizzle (not included in nutrition info:)

3 squares of a Lindt 90% chocolate bar

Instructions

For the crepes:

- Combine all of the crepes ingredients in a blender and blend until smooth.
- Let the batter rest for 5 minutes and then give it a stir to break up any additional air bubbles.
- Heat 1 teaspoon of butter in a 10 inch or larger nonstick saute pan over medium heat.
- When the butter is melted and bubbling, pour in about 1/4 cup of batter (you can eyeball it) and if necessary, gently tilt the pan in a circular motion to create a 6-inch (-ish) round crepe.
- Cook for two minutes, or until the top is no longer glossy and bubbles have formed almost to the middle of the crepe.
- Carefully flip and cook for another 30 seconds. Remove and place on a plate.
- Repeat until you have 8 usable crepes.

Nutrition Info

Serving Size: 2 stuffed crepes
Calories: 478
Fat: 42g
Carbohydrates: 4g
Fiber: 0g
Protein: 16g

Chocolate-Raspberry Chia Pudding Shots

Dessert and breakfast, together once more! These Chocolate-Raspberry Chia pudding shots are relatively similar to enchantment. They're solid and sweet - the ideal mix. Celebrated for being a low carb thickening agent, these natural chia seeds make a remarkable pudding!

Course: Breakfast, Dessert;
Prep Time 1 hour;
Servings 2; Calories 240 kcal

Ingredients:

- ¼ cup chia seeds
- 1/2 cup coconut milk
- 1/4 cup almond milk
- 1 tablespoon cacao powder
- 1 tablespoon Stevia
- 1/2 cup raspberries

Instructions:

- In a container, bring together all the ingredients (with the exception of the raspberries) and shake vivaciously. Let sit for 2 minutes and after that fill four shot glasses.

- Refrigerate for no less than 60 minutes (ideally across the night) until the point that blend thickens into pudding. Top with raspberries.

Recipe Notes:

This yield of this recipe is 4 shots. 1 serving is 2 shots.

Nutritional Information:
Calories: 241, Protein: 4g Fats: 20g, , Net Carbs: 4g

LUNCH

Keto Chicken Enchilada Bowl

This Keto Chicken Enchilada Bowl is a low carb twist on a Mexican favorite!

Prep Time: 20 minutes
Cook Time: 30 minutes
Total Time: 50 minutes
Yield: 4 servings

Ingredients

- 2 tablespoons coconut oil (for searing chicken)
- 1 pound of boneless, skinless chicken thighs
- 3/4 cup red enchilada sauce (recipe from Low Carb Maven)
- 1/4 cup water
- 1/4 cup chopped onion
- 4 oz can diced green chiles

Toppings (feel free to customize)

- 1 whole avocado, diced
- 1 cup shredded cheese (I used mild cheddar)

- 1/4 cup chopped pickled jalapenos
- 1/2 cup sour cream
- 1 roma tomato, chopped

Optional: serve over plain cauliflower rice (or Mexican cauliflower rice) for a more complete meal!

Instructions

- In a pot or dutch oven over medium heat melt the coconut oil. Once hot, sear chicken thighs until lightly brown.

- Pour in enchilada sauce and water then add onion and green chiles. Reduce heat to a simmer and cover. Cook chicken for 17-25 minutes or until chicken is tender and fully cooked through to at least 165 degrees internal temperature.

- Carefully remove the chicken and place onto a work surface. Chop or shred chicken (your preference) then add it back into the pot. Let the chicken simmer uncovered for an additional 10 minutes to absorb flavor and allow the sauce to reduce a little.

- To Serve, top with avocado, cheese, jalapeno, sour cream, tomato, and any other desired toppings. Feel free to customize these to your preference. Serve alone or over cauliflower rice if desired just be sure to update your personal nutrition info as needed.

Nutrition Info

Calories: 568 Calories

Total Carbs: 10.41g

Fiber: 4.27g

Net Carbs: 6.14g

Protein: 38.38g

Fat: 40.21g

Almond Coconut Curry on Veges

This almond coconut curry is super speedy and simple and tastes extraordinary as well! It flaunts nutritious vegetables alongside solid fats and a decent calorie tally.

Time 15 minutes; Total Time 15 minutes; Servings 4; Calories 439 kcal

Ingredients:

For the veges
For the curry

- 1 tsp coconut oil
- 400 ml coconut milk
- 2 cups mushrooms
- 125 g almond butter (100% ground almonds)
- 4 cups spinach
- 1 tbsp tomato paste
- 2 cups brocolli (chopped into florets)
- 1 tbsp curry powder

Instructions:

For the curry mixture

- Put the coconut drain, almond spread, tomato glue and curry powder in a blender. Mix for around 20 seconds or until smooth.
- Add the curry blend to a pan on low-medium warmth and warmth for 10-15 minutes or until warmed through. Blend habitually to abstain from staying.

For the veges

- Heat the coconut oil in a container on medium-high warmth and include the broccoli and mushrooms. Sear for around 3 minutes. Include the spinach and warmth for one more moment.

- Serve the veges in a bowl with the curry blend poured over the best.

Recipe Notes:

You can make the almond margarine by granulating almonds in a sustenance processor.

The curry blend isolates whenever left to sit in the refrigerator for some time, so make certain to mix it completely before utilizing on the off chance that you have put away it in the ice chest.

Nutritional Information:
Calories: 438, Fats: 41g, Protein: 11g, Net Carbs: 9g

Sesame Salmon w. Baby Bok Choy & Mushrooms

Ingredients

Main Dish

- 4 each 4-6 oz. salmon fillet
- 2 each portobello mushroom caps (or 8 oz. baby bella mushrooms)
- 4 each baby bok choy
- 1 tbsp toasted sesame seeds
- 1 ea green onion

Marinade

- 1 tbsp olive oil
- 1 tsp sesame oil
- 1 tbsp Coconut Aminos
- 1/2 inch Ginger grated (approx. 1 tsp.)
- 1/2 lemon juice
- 1/2 tsp Salt
- 1/2 tsp black pepper

Instructions

- Whisk together all of your marinade ingredients
- Drizzle half of the marinade on the salmon and turn to coat. Cover and refrigerate the salmon while it marinates for one hour.
- Preheat oven to 400.
- Prepare vegetables: Trim the rough ends from the bok choy and cut into halves. Slice the mushrooms into ½ inch pieces.
- Drizzle the remaining marinade over the vegetables and lay on a lined baking sheet.
- Place salmon, skin side down, on a lined baking sheet as well. Bake until salmon is cooked through, about 20 minutes.
- Top with sliced green onions and sesame seeds.

Caprese Tuna Salad Stuffed Tomatoes

Prep Time: 10 minutes
Yield: Serves 1
Serving Size: entire recipe
Calories per serving: 196
Fat per serving: 4.9g

Ingredients

- 1 medium tomato
- 1 (5oz) can tuna, very well drained
- 2 tsp balsamic vinegar
- 1 TBSP chopped mozzarella {1/4 oz.}
- 1 TBSP chopped fresh basil
- 1 TBSP chopped green onion

Instructions

- Cut the top 1/4-inch off the tomato. Use a spoon to scoop out the insides of the tomato. Set aside while you make the tuna salad.
- Stir together the drained tuna, balsamic vinegar, mozzarella, basil, and green onion. Put the tuna salad in the hollowed out tomato, and enjoy!
- Note: I prefer using fresh mozzarella but any mozzarella is good in here.

Salmon & Avocado Nori Rolls (Paleo Sushi)

Prep time: 10 mins
Total time: 10 mins
Recipe type: Lunch
Serves: 1

Ingredients

- 3 square nori sheets (seaweed wrappers)
- 150-180 g / 5-6 oz cooked salmon or tinned salmon
- ⅓ red pepper, sliced into thin strips
- ½ avocado, sliced into strips
- ½ small cucumber, sliced into strips
- 1 spring onion/scallion, cut into 2-3" pieces
- 2 tablespoons mayonnaise
- 1 tablespoon hot sauce or Sriracha sauce
- 1 teaspoon black or white sesame seeds
- Coconut aminos for dipping, optional

Instructions

- Place the nori sheet on a flat surface, such as a cutting board, shiny side down. Look at the fibres of the wrapper to see which way it needs to be rolled.
- Add a third of the salmon to the right or left third of the nori sheet and top with two strips of pepper, cucumber and avocado. Add some green onion and a drizzle of mayonnaise and hot sauce. You can sprinkle with sesame seeds now or at a later stage, once the rolls are cut.
- Lightly wet the top part of the nori sheet (the side you are rolling towards), just 1-2 cm of the wrapper. Pick up the opposite outer edge of the roll and start wrapping it over the ingredients, using your fingers to keep it nice and tight. This can take a bit of practice, but don't worry if your roll doesn't look perfect. Roll it until the top edge of the wrapper overlaps the roll and press it tightly to stick. Place the roll on the cutting board with the seam facing down and then cut into bite-size pieces.
- Scrve right away with some coconut aminos or extra mayo for dipping, or pack in a container to take for lunch or keep as a snack in the fridge.

Cinnamon Pork Chops & Mock Apples

Hearty, healthy, and delicious, cinnamon pork chops with chayote mock apples makes a fantastic family dinner or meal prep for the work week!

Prep Time 5 minutes
Cook Time 40 minutes
Total Time 45 minutes

Ingredients

- 2 tbsp ghee
- 1/2 tsp sea salt
- 4 pork chops boneless
- 2 chayote chopped to 1/2-inch chunks
- 2 tbsp monkfruit sweetener or low carb sweetener of choice
- 1 tsp cinnamon
- 1/8 tsp nutmeg
- 1 tbsp apple cider vinegar

Instructions

- Melt ghee in a large skillet over medium heat, add pork chops and cook for 5 minutes.

- Flip the pork chops and add chayote and sprinkle sweetener, cinnamon, nutmeg, and apple cider vinegar over the top. Cook for an additional 4-5 minutes, or until the pork chops reach the appropriate temperature (145 F for medium rare, 160 for medium).

- Remove the pork chops and place in a meal prep container if preparing meals for the week, otherwise keep pork chops warm until ready to serve.

- Bring the chayote mixture to a boil for several minutes. Reduce heat to low medium and simmer with cover, stirring occasionally, for 30 to 40 minutes. When done, the chayote will be fork tender and similar in texture to baked apple.

- Divide the chayote mock apples between four meal prep containers or serve immediately alongside the warm pork chops.

Recipe Notes

2g net carbohydrates per serving - which gives you room for a couple more things if you'd like to add that to your meal prep container or tailor things to your personal macros.

Nutritional Information:

Net Carbs: 4.85g
Protein: 35.43g
Fat: 30.22g
Calories: 455kcal

Loaded Chicken Salad

A delicious salad filled with plenty of vegetables and delicious grilled meat!

Prep Time 10 minutes
Cook Time 8 minutes
Total Time 18 minutes
Total Carbs 12.86g

Ingredients

- 1 boneless chicken breast (about 300g, with or without skin)
- 1 tbsp extra virgin olive oil
- 1/4 tsp Himalayan salt
- 1/4 tsp black pepper
- 1 avocado
- 100 g mozzarella balls
- 1 large tomato (any colour)
- 1 har artichoke hearts (my jar was 170g)
- 1/2 red onion
- 5 asparagus
- 20 leaves basil
- 4 cups baby spinach (200g used)

Dressing

- 2 tbsp extra virgin olive oil
- 1 1/2 tbsp balsamic vinegar
- 1 tsp dijon mustard
- 1 clove garlic
- pinch Himalayan salt
- pinch black pepper

Instructions

- Peel and dice the avocado. Slice the red onion. Dice the tomato. Pile the basil leaves together, roll them up and slice. Cut the stems off the asparagus and slice in half. Mince the garlic.
- Slice the chicken breast in half lengthwise. Sprinkle the 1/4 tsp of salt and pepper on each sides. Heat the 1 tbsp of olive oil in a cast iron skillet and place the chicken breasts in. Fry on each side, about 3 minutes each side, until they have a nice golden brown colour and cooked through. Add the asparagus beside the chicken breasts and cook a few minutes until soft and grilled. Take out the chicken and slice.

- In a small bowl, combine the minced garlic, olive oil, balsamic vinegar, dijon, and salt & pepper.
- Add the baby spinach to a large bowl or plate. Cover with the grilled chicken, avocado, mozzarella, tomatoes, artichoke, red onions, asparagus and basil leaves. Pour the dressing over and enjoy!

Notes

You can add 1 tbsp of honey to the salad dressing if you don't mind the extra carbs or want a sweeter dressing.

Nutrition Info
Calories 430 Calories from Fat 264
Saturated Fat 6.57g 33%
Total Carbohydrates 12.86g 4%
Dietary Fiber 6.12g 24%
Sugars 3.16g
Protein 31.73g 63%

Dinner and Desert

Keto Instant Pot Crack Chicken Recipe

Cuisine: American
Prep time: 5 mins
Cook time: 20 mins
Total time: 25 mins
Serves: 8 servings (yields about 7 cups total)

Rich, creamy, and full of flavor, this Keto Instant Pot Crack Chicken Recipe is sure to be a favorite family dinner.

Ingredients

- 2 slices bacon, chopped
- 2 lbs (910 g) boneless, skinless chicken breasts
- 2 (8 oz/227 g) blocks cream cheese
- ½ cup (120 ml) water
- 2 tablespoons apple cider vinegar
- 1 tablespoon dried chives
- 1½ teaspoons garlic powder
- 1½ teaspoons onion powder
- 1 teaspoon crushed red pepper flakes

- 1 teaspoon dried dill
- ¼ teaspoon salt
- ¼ teaspoon black pepper
- ½ cup (2 oz/57 g) shredded cheddar
- 1 scallion, green and white parts, thinly sliced

Instructions

- Turn pressure cooker on, press "Sauté", and wait 2 minutes for the pot to heat up. Add the chopped bacon and cook until crispy. Transfer to a plate and set aside. Press "Cancel" to stop sautéing.
- Add the chicken, cream cheese, water, vinegar, chives, garlic powder, onion powder, crushed red pepper flakes, dill, salt, and black pepper to the pot. Turn the pot on Manual, High Pressure for 15 minutes and then do a Quick release.
- Use tongs to transfer the chicken to a large plate, shred it with 2 forks, and return it back to the pot.
- Stir in the cheddar cheese.
- Top with the crispy bacon and scallion, and serve.

Notes

We've tested this recipe upwards of 10 times and have never had the burn warning come on; however, several readers have had the warning come on, so we want to give a tip. In step 1 of the Instructions above, after removing the bacon from the pot, we recommend adding a splash of water, and use a wooden spoon to scrape up any brown bits that have formed on the bottom to deglaze the pan. After that, continue on with step 1 and press "Cancel" to stop sauteing.

Nutrition Facts

Calories: 437 Fat: 27.6 Potassium: 390 Net Carbs: 4.3 Carbohydrates: 4.5 Sodium: 420 Fiber: .2 Protein: 41.2

Keto Chicken Enchilada Bowl

This Keto Chicken Enchilada Bowl is a low carb twist on a Mexican favorite! It's So easy to make, totally filling and ridiculously yummy!

Prep Time: 20 minutes
Cook Time: 30 minutes
Total Time: 50 minutes
Yield: 4 servings

Ingredients

- 2 tablespoons coconut oil (for searing chicken)
- 1 pound of boneless, skinless chicken thighs
- 3/4 cup red enchilada sauce (recipe from Low Carb Maven)
- 1/4 cup water
- 1/4 cup chopped onion
- 4 oz can diced green chiles

Toppings (feel free to customize)

- 1 whole avocado, diced
- 1 cup shredded cheese (I used mild cheddar)
- 1/4 cup chopped pickled jalapenos

- 1/2 cup sour cream
- 1 roma tomato, chopped

Optional: serve over plain cauliflower rice (or mexican cauliflower rice) for a more complete meal!

Instructions

- In a pot or dutch oven over medium heat melt the coconut oil. Once hot, sear chicken thighs until lightly brown.

- Pour in enchilada sauce and water then add onion and green chiles. Reduce heat to a simmer and cover. Cook chicken for 17-25 minutes or until chicken is tender and fully cooked through to at least 165 degrees internal temperature.

- Careully remove the chicken and place onto a work surface. Chop or shred chicken (your preference) then add it back into the pot. Let the chicken simmer uncovered for an additional 10 minutes to absorb flavor and allow the sauce to reduce a little.

- To Serve, top with avocado, cheese, jalapeno, sour cream, tomato, and any other desired toppings. Feel free to customize these to your preference. Serve alone or over cauliflower rice if desired just be sure to update your personal nutrition info as needed.

Nutrition Info

Calories: 568 Calories
Total Carbs: 10.41g
Fiber: 4.27g
Net Carbs: 6.14g
Protein: 38.38g
Fat: 40.21g

Crab Stuffed Mushrooms With Cream Cheese

An easy recipe for crab stuffed mushrooms with cream cheese. Low carb, keto, and gluten free.

Prep Time 15 minutes
Cook Time 30 minutes
Servings 4 servings
Calories 160 kcal

Ingredients

- 20 ounces cremini (baby bella) mushrooms (20-25 individual mushrooms)
- 2 tablespoons finely grated parmesan cheese
- 1 tablespoon chopped fresh parsley
- salt

Filling:

- 4 ounces cream cheese softened to room temperature
- 4 ounces crab meat finely chopped
- 5 cloves garlic minced
- 1 teaspoon dried oregano
- 1/2 teaspoon paprika

- 1/2 teaspoon black pepper
- 1/4 teaspoon salt

Instructions

- Preheat the oven to 400 F. Prepare a baking sheet lined with parchment paper.
- Snap stems from mushrooms, discarding the stems and placing the mushroom caps on the baking sheet 1 inch apart from each other. Season the mushroom caps with salt.
- In a large mixing bowl, combine all filling ingredients and stir until well-mixed without any lumps of cream cheese. Stuff the mushroom caps with the mixture. Evenly sprinkle parmesan cheese on top of the stuffed mushrooms.
- Bake at 400 F until the mushrooms are very tender and the stuffing is nicely browned on top, about 30 minutes. Top with parsley and serve while hot.

Nutrition Notes

This recipe yields 5 g net carbs per serving (5-6 stuffed mushrooms).

Nutrition Info

Calories 160

Total Carb 5.5g 2%

Dietary Fiber 0.5g 1%

Sugars 0g

Protein 9g

Lemon Butter Sauce for Fish

Prep: 5 mins
Cook: 10 mins
Total: 15 mins

A Lemon Butter Sauce with Crispy Pan Fried Fish that would be perfectly at home in a posh restaurant, yet is so quick to make at home! Browning the butter gives the sauce a rich, nutty aroma which pairs beautifully with fresh lemon, as well as thickening the sauce and giving it a gorgeous golden colour. Recipe VIDEO below (helpful for pre-post browned butter).

Servings: 2
Calories: 393 kcal

Ingredients

Lemon Butter Sauce:

- 60 g / 4 tbsp unsalted butter, cut into pieces
- 1 tbsp fresh lemon juice
- Salt and finely ground pepper

Crispy Pan Fried Fish:

- 2 x thin white fish fillets (120-150g / 4-5oz each), skinless boneless (I used Bream, Note 1)
- Salt and pepper
- 2 tbsp white flour
- 2 tbsp oil (I use canola)

Serving:

- Lemon wedges
- Finely chopped parsley, optional

Instructions

- Lemon Butter Sauce (see video):

- Place the butter in a light coloured saucepan or small skillet over medium heat.

- Melt butter then leave on the stove, whisking / stirring very now and then. When the butter turns golden brown and it smells nutty - about 3 minutes, remove from stove immediately and pour into small bowl. (Note 2)

- Add lemon juice and a pinch of salt and pepper. Stir then taste when it has cooled slightly. Adjust lemon/salt to taste.

- Set aside - it will stay pourable for 20 - 30 minutes. See Note 3 for storing.

Crispy Pan Fried Fish:

- Pat fish dry using paper towels. Sprinkle with salt & pepper, then flour. Use fingers to spread flour. Turn and repeat. Shake excess flour off well, slapping between hands if necessary.

- Heat oil in a nonstick skillet over high heat. When the oil is shimmering and there are faint wisps of smoke, add fish. Cook for 1 1/2 minutes until golden and crispy on the edges, then turn and cook the other side for 1 1/2 minutes (cook longer if you have thicker fillets).

- Remove immediately onto serving plates. Drizzle each with about 1 tbsp of Sauce (avoid dark specks settled at the bottom of the bowl), garnish with parsley and serve with lemon on the side. Pictured in post with Kale and Quinoa Salad.

Recipe Notes

If you're an experienced cook, you can try your hand at making the sauce in the pan after cooking the fish. First wipe it clean (yes you lose pan flavour, but it's nice to have a "clean" looking sauce), lower heat then make the sauce once the pan has cooled. I personally find it easier to make the Sauce first in a smaller pan - easier to control colour change. Also I like using my black non stick pan for the fish and you can't see the colour of the butter in dark coloured pans.

Easy Tomato Feta Soup Recipe

Prep Time:5 mins
Cook Time:25 mins
Total Time:30 mins
Servings: 6

Easy Tomato Feta Soup Recipe - Low Calorie, Low Carb, Keto - simple to make with just a few simple basic ingredients. Creamy tomato soup with basil and rich, savory feta cheese. Ready on 30 minutes on the stove top.

Ingredients

- 2 tbsp olive oil or butter
- 1/4 cup chopped onion
- 2 cloves garlic
- 1/2 tsp salt
- 1/8 tsp black pepper
- 1 tsp pesto sauce — optional
- 1/2 tsp dried oregano
- 1 tsp dried basil
- 1 tbsp tomato paste — optional
- 10 tomatoes, skinned, seeded and chopped — or two 14.5 oz cans of peeled tomatoes
- 1 tsp honey, sugar or erythritol — optional
- 3 cups water
- 1/3 cup heavy cream
- 2/3 cup feta cheese — crumbled

Instructions

- Heat olive oil (butter) over medium heat in a large pot (Dutch Oven). Add the onion and cook for 2 minutes, stirring freɋuently. Add the garlic and cook for 1 minute. Add tomatoes, salt, pepper, pesto (optional), oregano, basil, tomato paste and water. Bring to a boil, then reduce to a simmer. Add sweetener.

- Cook on medium heat for 20 minutes, until the tomatoes are tender and cooker. Using an immersion blender, blend until smooth. Add the cream and feta cheese. Cook for 1 more minute.

- Add more salt if needed. Serve warm.

Recipe Notes

For people who are against using heavy cream in keto diet, you can use almond milk.

Nutrition Information

Calories: 170, Fat: 13g, Saturated Fat: 8g, Cholesterol: 43mg, Sodium: 464mg, Potassium: 542mg, Carbohydrates: 10g, Fiber: 2g, Sugar: 6g, Protein: 4g, Vitamin A: 43%, Vitamin C: 35.7%, Calcium: 11.9%, Iron: 4.9%

Instant Pot Beef Bourguignon

Instant Pot Beef Bourguignon is a pressure cooker recipe with beef, mushrooms, onions, and carrots cooked in red wine. Low carb, keto, and gluten free.

Prep Time 30 minutes
Cook Time 50 minutes
Servings 6 servings
Calories 220 kcal

Ingredients

- 1.5 - 2 pounds beef chuck roast cut into 3/4-inch cubes
- 5 strips bacon diced
- 1 small onion chopped
- 10 ounces cremini mushrooms quartered
- 2 carrots chopped
- 5 cloves garlic minced
- 3 bay leaves
- 3/4 cup dry red wine
- 3/4 teaspoon xanthan gum (or corn starch, read post for instructions)
- 1 tablespoon tomato paste
- 1 teaspoon dried thyme
- salt & pepper

Instructions

- Generously season beef chunks with salt and pepper, and set aside. Select the saute mode on the pressure cooker for medium heat. When the display reads HOT, add diced bacon and cook for about 5 minutes until crispy, stirring frequently. Transfer the bacon to a paper towel lined plate.

- Add the beef to the pot in a single layer and cook for a few minutes to brown, then flip and repeat for the other side. Transfer to a plate when done.

- Add onions and garlic. Cook for a few minutes to soften, stirring frequently. Add red wine and tomato paste, using a wooden spoon to briefly scrape up flavorful brown bits stuck to the bottom of the pot. Stir to check that the tomato paste is dissolved. Turn off the saute mode.

- Transfer the beef back to the pot. Add mushrooms, carrots, and thyme, stirring together. Top with bay leaves. Secure and seal the lid. Cook at high pressure for 40 minutes, followed by a manual pressure release.

- Uncover and select the saute mode. Remove bay leaves. Evenly sprinkle xanthan gum over the pot and stir together. Let the stew boil for a minute to thicken while stirring. Turn off the saute mode. Serve into bowls and top with crispy bacon.

Nutrition Notes

This recipe yields 5.5 g net carbs per serving (1-1.5 cups).

Nutrition Info

Calories 220

Total Fat 5g 8%

Sodium 310mg 13%

Potassium 130mg 4%

Total Carb 6.5g 2%

Dietary Fiber 1g 3%

Sugars 2g

Protein 27g

Keto Chicken Pot Pie

Cook Time22 mins
Course: Main Course
Servings: 8 servings
Calories: 297kcal

Ingredients

For the Chicken Pot Pie Filling:

- 2 tablespoons of butter
- 1/2 cup mixed veggies could also substitute green beans or broccoli
- 1/4 small onion diced
- 1/4 tsp pink salt
- 1/4 tsp pepper
- 2 garlic cloves minced
- 3/4 cup heavy whipping cream
- 1 cup chicken broth
- 1 tsp poultry seasoning
- 1/4 tsp rosemary
- pinch thyme
- 2 1/2 cups cooked chicken diced
- 1/4 tsp Xanthan Gum

For the crust:

- 4 1/2 tablespoons of butter melted and cooled
- 1/3 cup coconut flour
- 2 tablespoons full fat sour cream
- 4 eggs
- 1/4 teaspoon salt
- 1/4 teaspoon baking powder
- 1 1/3 cup sharp shredded cheddar cheese or mozzarella shredded

Instructions

- Cook 1 to 1 1/2 lbs chicken in the slow cooker for 3 hours on high or 6 hours on low.
- Preheat oven to 400 degrees.
- Sautee onion, mixed veggies, garlic cloves, salt, and pepper in 2 tablespoons butter in an oven safe skillet for approx 5 min or until onions are translucent.
- Add heavy whipping cream, chicken broth, poultry seasoning, thyme, and rosemary.
- Sprinkle Xanthan Gum on top and simmer for 5 minutes so that the sauce thickens. Make sure to simmer covered as the liquid will evaporate otherwise. You need a lot of

liquid for this recipe, otherwise, it will be dry.

- Add diced chicken.
- Make the breading by combining melted butter (I cool mine by popping the bowl in the fridge for 5 min), eggs, salt, and sour cream in a bowl then whisk together.
- Add coconut flour and baking powder to the mixture and stir until combined.
- Stir in cheese.
- Drop batter by dollops on top of the chicken pot pie. Do not spread it out, as the coconut flour will absorb too much of the liquid.
- Bake in a 400-degree oven for 15-20 min.
- Set oven to broil and move chicken pot pie to top shelf. Broil for 1-2 minutes until bread topping is nicely browned.

Nutrition

Calories: 297kcal | Carbohydrates: 5.3g | Protein: 11.6g | Fat: 17g | Fiber: 2g

Easy Stir Fry Kimchi & Pork Belly

Stir-fry kimchi and bork belly is so simple to make yet out of this world satisfying! Dinner under 30 minutes, and Keto friendly.

Prep Time5 mins
Cook Time: 15 mins
Marinating: Time10 mins
Total Time: 20 mins
Servings: 3 people
Calories: 804 kcal

Ingredients

- 300 g naturally-raised pork belly
- 1 tbsp naturally-brewed tamari or soy sauce (gluten-free option: use tamari or gluten-free soy sauce)
- 1 tbsp naturally-brewed rice wine
- 1 lb kimchi (see notes below)
- 1 stalk green onion
- 1 tbsp sesame seeds (optional)

Instructions

- Slice the pork belly as thin as possible. Marinate in tamari/soy sauce and rice wine for about 10 minutes. If your kimchi isn't pre-cut, then cut into 1 inch size.

- Heat a heavy bottom pan (I use cast iron). While the pan is very hot, add the marinated pork belly, stir fry until nicely browned, for approximately 5 to 10 minutes. You should see some fat being cooked out of the pork belly at this point.

- Add the kimchi into the pan, stir-fry for another 2 minutes, for the flavour of kimchi and pork to completely mix.

- Turn off the heat. Thinly slice the green onion, and add to the stir fry.

- If available, sprinkle sesame seeds on top as garnish.

Recipe Notes

If you use a store-bought kimchi, make sure to check the ingredients. I use a home-made fermented kimchi that's free of MSG and added sugar (recipe coming soon.)

Spinach Artichoke Stuffed Chicken Breast Recipe

Spinach Artichoke Stuffed Chicken Breast is the perfect combination of your favorite dip and favorite bird, all rolled into one quick and easy Ketogenic stuffed chicken breast recipe! These spinach and mozzarella stuffed chicken breasts are gluten-free, low-carb, and Keto diet-approved!

Prep Time 15 minutes
Cook Time 15 minutes
Total Time 30 minutes
Servings 6 servings
Calories 288 kcal

Ingredients

- 1 ½ lbs. chicken breasts 6 4-oz. portions
- 2 tablespoons olive oil
- 4 ounces cream cheese softened
- ¼ cup Greek yogurt
- ½ cup Mozzarella cheese shredded
- ½ cup artichoke hearts thinly sliced
- ¼ cup frozen spinach drained, and tightly packed
- ½ tsp. salt divided
- ¼ tsp. pepper divided

Instructions

- Pound chicken breast to 1-inch thick. Using a sharp knife cut each chicken breast down the middle, being careful not to cut all of the way through, to make a pocket for the spinach artichoke filling. Sprinkle chicken breasts with ¼ teaspoon salt and 1/8 teaspoon pepper.
- In a medium-sized bowl combine the cream cheese, Greek yogurt, Mozzarella cheese, artichoke hearts, drained spinach, ¼ teaspoon salt and 1/8 teaspoon pepper. Mix until thoroughly combined.
- Carefully fill each chicken breast with equal amounts of the spinach artichoke filling. If you have extra filling, set it aside until the chicken is almost done cooking.
- In a large skillet over medium heat add olive oil and stuffed chicken breasts. Cover skillet and cook for 7-8 minutes on each side, or until chicken reaches 165 degrees with a meat thermometer.
- During the last few minutes of cooking, add additional filling to the skillet to heat it up. Serve chicken with cauliflower rice, regular rice, mashed cauliflower, or mashed potatoes and enjoy!

Nutrition Facts

Calories 288 Calories from Fat 153
Total Fat 17g 26%
Total Carbohydrates 2g 1%
Sugars 1g

CONCLUSION

The keto plan is a versatile and interesting way to lose weight, with lots of delicious food choices. Keep these 10 items stocked in your fridge, freezer, and larder, and you'll be ready to throw together some delicious keto meals and snacks at a moment's notice.

KETO VEGAN

Low Carb Diet Recipes For Weight Loss, Burn Fat, Boost Your Energy.

Holly R.Evans

TABLE OF CONTENTS

PART ONE: THE KETO-VEGAN LIFESTYLE

PART TWO: THE 7-DAY MEAL PLAN

PART THREE: PUTTING IT ALL TOGETHER

BREAKFAST

LUNCH

DINNER

PART FOUR: CONCLUSION

INTRODUCTION

The keto-vegan diet is a food guideline that comprises of low carbohydrates, moderate protein content and are rich in fats and oils. It became very popular over the years because of its tremendous efficiency on weight loss programs and general wellbeing. While the parent keto diet often has to do with animal foods, keto-vegan is based primarily on plant foods while still maintaining the original macro content ratios. Pure vegan diets is devoid of any animal product and as a result, it becomes increasingly difficult to consume low carbohydrate. The good news is, with careful planning of keto-vegan meals, vegans can as well benefit from the health promoting effects of a ketogenic diets. This work succinctly explains not just what to include and what to avoid in a well-planned ketogenic diet, it can also serve as a complete guide to anyone willing to adopt the keto-vegan dietary program and also provides a 7 days keto-vegan meal plan and recipes.

PART ONE

THE KETO-VEGAN LIFESTYLE

CHAPTER 1

Keto-vegan Diet Guide:

The keto-vegan diet is a food guideline that comprises of low carbohydrates, moderate protein content and are rich in fats and oils. It became very popular over the years because of its tremendous efficiency on weight loss programs and general wellbeing. While the parent keto diet often has to do with animal foods, keto-vegan is based primarily on plant foods while still maintaining the original macro content ratios. Pure vegan diets is devoid of any animal product and as a result, it becomes increasingly difficult to consume low carbohydrate. The good news is, with careful planning of keto-vegan meals, vegans can as well benefit from the health promoting effects of a ketogenic diets. This work succinctly explains not just what to include and what to avoid in a well-planned ketogenic diet, it can also serve as a complete guide to anyone willing to adopt the keto-vegan dietary program and also provides a 7 days keto-vegan meal plan and recipes.

What Is the Keto-vegan Diet?

The keto-vegan diet comprises of foods that are low in carbohydrate content, contains moderate amounts of protein and are very rich (up to 80%) in fats and oils. In a typical keto-vegan meal, carbohydrates are drastically reduced to not even up to 50 grams per day. This is to enable the body reach and maintain a metabolic state called KETOSIS which is the goal of every ketogenic diet. Due to the fact that this dietary guideline is basically made of fats for the most part – somewhere around 80% of whole food – keto-vegans turn to high-oil plant products like avocado, olive, and coconut, making it possible for vegans, to also follow a ketogenic dietary guideline as well.

The keto-Vegan diet comprises of moderate protein content, low carbohydrate, and is rich in fats and does not include any food of animal origin but plants.

People on a vegan dietary guideline only take in food products of plant origin like grains, vegetables, and fruits and avoid any food of animal product like dairy, meats and poultry. Vegans are able to achieve and maintaining ketosis by subsisting on plant-based foods that are rich in fats content such as olive oil, coconut oil and avocados.

WHY LOW-CARB, HIGH-FAT?

EATING A HIGH FAT, LOW-CARBOHYDRATE DIET is important for every weight loss campaign. Even more importantly, findings from an increasing number of empirical researches shows that high-fat, low-carb foods help reduce an individual's chances and risks of coming down with systemic illnesses like heart disorders, diabetes, stroke or apoplexy, epilepsy and Alzheimer's. The keto-vegan dietary guideline promotes the consumption of fresh, organic whole foods like vegetables and fruits, and nourishing oils of plant origin. It's a dietary guideline with a long-term sustainability potential and is also enjoyable.

Carbohydrates (sugar) brings about blood glucose sky-rocketing, which leads to crashes almost immediately, and then the accompanying cravings for more carbohydrates and sugars. This dangerous cascade of events leads to consistent spikes in insulin and the accompanying pre-diabetes and diabetes type II.

Research findings consistently indicate that keto-vegan dietary guidelines enable people lose more pounds, causes improved energy levels for daily activities, curbs cravings and promotes long durations of satiety. The ability to curb cravings and promote satiety for long durations is because most of the caloric content in a keto-vegan diet originates from fat which is calorically dense and is slow in digestion. This makes it typical for keto-vegan eaters to consume lesser calories.

CHAPTER 2

Why Go Keto-Vegan?

Consuming and maintaining a keto-vegan diet turns your body into an efficient machine for burning fat for metabolic fuel or energy. This is actually fantastic for a good number of reasons, not just that fats contains 2 times as much calories as carbohydrates, making you eat twice as less food by weight every day, the body attains a better position to get rid of stored fats (which a lot of people try so hard to burn) resulting in loss of more pounds. Making use of fats as a substrate for metabolic fuel ensures a consistent energy level for daily activities and the good news is, it does not mess with the blood glucose levels, thus with keto-vegan diets, you don't have to experience the lows and lows associated with consuming carbohydrates in high amounts. Consistent energy levels for the whole day means you can achieve more and as a matter of fact, feel less tired doing more.

In addition to the benefits highlighted above, consuming and maintaining keto-vegan diets for long can:

- Maintain steady levels of HDL (good) and LDL (bad) cholesterol
- Bring about more weight loss (specifically body fat)
- Decrease blood sugar and insulin resistance
- Improve brain function
- Decrease triglyceride levels
- Decrease blood pressure

SUPPORT FOR YOUR NEW LIFESTYLE

When commencing the keto-vegan dietary program, it's very vital to let your family and closest friends or workplace colleagues to know you mean business concerning your new way of life and also detail them on the foods you need to stop eating. This has been proven to add strength to your support system as you will find helpful during social outings and gatherings like dinner and the rest. It's absolutely normal to be met with some resistance and challenges on start-up. Keep in mind that the high-fat, low-carb dietary guidelines has been the living standard in the lives of many people and keto-vegan is a complete turn of events. Just focus on yourself and the lifestyle goals you want to achieve. Sooner than you'll realize, your low levels of energy, reduction in body weight, and improved outlook will leave even naysayers wondering.

One awesome place where you can start building your support system is reddit.com's keto-vegan sub reddit: www.reddit.com/r/keto-vegan

You'll discover numerous other keto-veganers from all around the globe sharing their experiences and progress notes, and also supporting others in this journey of complete turnaround.

Getting into Ketosis

When you are consuming and maintaining a diet that's rich in carbohydrate, your body is in a metabolic status known as glycolysis (sugar breakdown). The simple implication is that most of the metabolic fuel or energy your body uses for daily activities originates from blood glucose content. In this condition, immediately after each meal consumption, your blood glucose is sharply increased bringing about lower body insulin levels, and ths shortage in insulin drives the storage of body fat and also inhibits or prevents the release of fats from their storage sites (adipose tissues) in the body.

However, when you consume and maintain a low-carbohydrate, high-fat diet, the reverse becomes the case. Your body attains a metabolic condition known as KETOSIS. In this status, your body readily and efficiently breaks down fat into ketone bodies (ketones) for metabolic fuel as its primary energy source and fats storage sites are consistently emptied. It's a biologically normal state and you're not overriding anything as naysayers may think—as a matter of fact, whenever you consume low carbohydrate than your body requires, your body falls back to this status naturally.

WHAT TO DO IF YOU HAVE DIABETES

The good news for persons with type 2 diabetes is that the keto-vegan low-carb, high-fat foods can start to kick in the diabetes condition in reverse gear. For type 1 diabetes, keto b-vegan can tremendously improve the body's control of blood glucose levels. Be sure to seek the counsel of your physician before embarking on any dietary guideline especially one that has to do with low carbohydrates intake. This is because if you take medications for diabetes type 1 for instance and want to embark on a low carbohydrate diet, it may become necessary and appropriate to reduce your dosages immediately. Your physician may recommend or suggest you embark on a period of trial or probation with your dietary guideline while he/she supervises. By so doing, they can maintain a close supervision on your blood glucose levels and insulin dosages. In addition, it is advisable to consume more than 50 grams of carbohydrate every day to prevent ketoacidosis in type 1 diabetes.

TESTING FOR KETOSIS

As soon as you commence your low-carb keto-vegan diet, one thing you should know is when and if you have achieved the state of ketosis. Not only does it help in increasing your confidence levels on the journey, testing your ketosis status helps you know you're on the right track and whether there's need to make some changes.

One very simple and easy test for ketosis is to sniff for "keto-breath." Few days from the moment you started eating low carb, it's normal for you to a fruity, metallic or even sour taste in your taste buds. This is because as soon as your body attains the state of ketosis, ketone bodies which are beta-hydroxybutyrate, acetoacetate and acetone are created in the body. Acetone is responsible for ketone breathe as it is excreted from the breath and the urine. Also, ketone urine test strips are also used to more accurately detect the presence of ketone bodies (acetone).

Similar to the USDA's Food Pyramid, the keto-vegan dietary guidelines is developed on macro ratios. It's very essential to obtain the appropriate macronutrients so as not to deprive your body of the energy it requires for daily activities and also of any essential dietary fat or protein. Macronutrients are carbohydrates, proteins and fats and are the major building blocks of the food we eat. Each one of the macros provides the body with a given amount of metabolic fuel or energy measure in calories per gram of macro eaten.

- **Fat = 9 calories per gram**
- **Protein = 4 calories per gram**
- **Carbohydrates = 4 calories per gram**

With the keto-vegan dietary guideline, about 75% percent of the calories intake is expected to be obtained from oils, while about 20 % is obtained from plant-based protein foods and the last 5% from carbohydrate foods of plant origin.

The number of calories you should eat depends on a few factors, including:

- **Current lean body weight**
- **The types of workouts**
- **Hours per week of each type**
- **Daily activity levels**
- **Gain muscle**
- **Maintain weight**
- **Workout regimen? If so:**
- **Goals**
- **Lose weight**

You can also find plenty of helpful tools for calculation with a quick Google search for "keto calculator." You'll be able to easily and quickly plug in your numbers and get an immediate estimation of your body's caloric needs.

One of the great things about the keto diet is that it's not necessary to track each and every number to hit your goals. Yet if you want to track, it's a great way to speed up your progress, and tracking will give you a visual reminder to stay on course every day.

Necessary Nutrients

It's crucial to drink plenty of water when beginning the

keto-vegan diet. In addition, it is also absolutely normal for you to be visiting the convenience more often. This happens because since you're drastically reducing your intake of processed or refined foods and have started eating organic and natural food products, you're also reducing your intake of certain minerals like sodium which is found in refined or processed foods so the abrupt dietary modification causes a sudden low in sodium intake.

More so, the sudden decrease in carbohydrate intake also reduces the level of insulin in the body, making the kidneys to release more sodium. As a result, the body removes more water through urine, causing you to urinate often and lose water and electrolytes.

When this is the case, the typical symptoms includes headaches, fatigue, nausea, and irritability.

This state is for the most part known as the "keto flu." It's imperative to realize this isn't the real influenza virus. It's known as the keto flu just because of the likeness in symptoms, however it's neither infectious nor a genuine virus.

Numerous people who encounter these symptoms trust the keto diet made them wiped out and promptly return to eating carbs. In any case, the keto flu stage really implies your body is pulling back from sugar, high carbs, and refined foods, and is straightening out so it can utilize fat as its fuel. The keto flu as a rule keeps going only a couple of days while the body rearranges. You can lessen its symptoms by adding more sodium and electrolytes to your eating regimen.

THE "KETO FLU"

The keto flu is avoidable and its duration can be reduced simply by adding more sodium to your diet. Here are some of the easiest ways to do it:

- Add more salt to your meals.
- Eat saltier foods like pickled vegetables and bacon.

Keto-vegan Weight Loss basics for Biggest Losers

1. **Check Out What Shape You're In**
   Start with a health check. See your GP and check out what shape your health is in, including blood pressure, cholesterol and blood sugar levels. Check your starting weight, waist and hip measurements. Write them down in a journal.

2. **Set A Weight Loss Goal**
   Start off by aiming to lose 5-10% of your starting weight. If you weigh 100 kilograms, aim to get to 90 kilograms over three to six months. Most people are not aware that losing this amoint of weight will reduce their risk of developing type 2 diabetes and greatly improve their health. Plus, it is a realistic goal.

3. **Get Organized**

    Get organized for a healthy Keto-vegan eating. This means you need to have a clean-up day in your kitchen! Get rid of all the junk foods and drinks lurking around in the panty, freezer and any secret hiding spot. Successful keto-vegan biggest losers plan their meal ahead of time. Plan out a whole week of meals in advance and then write out a matching grocery list. Do not buy foods that are not on the list or foods that do not belong there in a successful keto-vegan biggest loser's pantry, fridge or freezer.

4. **Make A Hobby Out Of Reading Food Labels.**

    Use the recipe and meal plan guide in this book to make over for your recipes in the keto-vegan biggest loser's style.

5. **Eat Your Way To Weight-Loss Healthy Living Success**

    Low carb, high fat meals turn keto-vegan biggest losers into weight loss winners. This means dramatically increasing your low carb vegetables, salads and fruits intake and also using the various forms of meat alternatives out there. Try a home delivery of fruits and vegetables service so that big quantities arrive automatically and give you an extra incentive to us emore of them. Plus it can be cheaper and the produce is delivered straight from the markets.

6. **Keep A Record Of What You Eat And How Active You Are**

   Every day, record what you eat and drink, as well as the physical activities and exercises you do. Use this information to work out which foods that provide most of your Calories and fat over bthe day. This is called self-monitoring. It keeps you honest about what you eat, ensuring you abide by the keto-vegan Do's and Don'ts. It also shows you how much exercise it will take to burn off your favorite treats and highlights how easily extra calories can sneak into your day.

Getting Ready to Go Keto-Vegan

Now that you understand the benefits and science behind the keto-vegan diet, you're ready to get started. In the following chapters, you'll get all the information you need to succeed with your keto-vegan diet, including what to buy and what to avoid, meal plans and full recipes, and physical activities or exercises to carry out to be in top health.

CHAPTER 3

GO KETO-VEGAN IN FIVE STEPS

Now that you've known the facts behind the low-carb high-fat keto-vegan dietary guidelines and why it does what you're about to experience. In this section, you'll figure out how to begin and amplify achievement. Here's a snappy and simple well-ordered manual for use as you start, and to allude to whenever all through your adventure, for help and direction.

Step 1: Clean Out Your Pantry

Out with the old, in with the new. Having tempting, unhealthy foods in your home is one of the biggest contributors to failure when starting any diet. To succeed, you need to minimize any triggers to maximize your chances. Unless you have the iron will of Arnold Schwarzenegger, you should not keep addictive foods like bread, desserts, and other non–keto friendly snacks around.

If you don't live alone, be sure to discuss and warn your housemates, whether they're significant others, family, or roommates. If some items must be kept (if they're simply not yours to throw out), try to agree on a special location to keep them out of sight. This will also help anyone you share your living space with understand that you are serious about starting your diet, and will lead to a better experience for you at home overall (people love to tempt anyone on a diet at first, but it will get old and they'll tire quickly).

STARCHES AND GRAINS
Do away with all high carbohydrate food like pasta, rice,

potatoes, bread, corns, bagels, oats, and croissants.

SUGARY FOODS AND DRINKS

Do away with all refined sugar foods and drinks like fruit juices, fountain drinks, fruit juices, pastries, candy bars, etc.

LEGUMES

Do away with beans, lentils, and peas. They are rich in carbohydrate contents. A 1-cup serving of beans alone provides more than triple of your daily carbohydrate allowance on a low-carb high-fat diet.

PROCESSED POLYUNSATURATED FATS AND OILS

Get rid of all vegetable oils and most seed oils, including sunflower, safflower, canola, soybean, grapeseed, and corn oil.

Also eliminate trans fats like shortening and margarine—anything that says "hydrogenated" or "partially hydrogenated." Olive oil, extra-virgin olive oil, avocado oil, and coconut oil are the keto-vegan-friendly oils you want on hand.

FRUITS

Get rid of fruits that are high in carbs, including bananas, dates, grapes, mangos, and apples. Be sure to get rid of any dried fruits like raisins as well. Dried fruit contains as much sugar as regular fruit but more concentrated, making it easy to eat a lot of sugar in a small serving. For comparison, a cup of raisins has over 100 grams of carbs while a cup of grapes has only 15 grams of carbs.

Yes, you're "getting rid" of unwanted foods in your pantry, but these foods can feed many others. Please, don't throw them away! Find a local food bank or homeless youth shelter to donate them to.Your pantry will seem empty after the cleanout. That's because products meant for longer-term storage are usually high in carbs and full of unhealthy additives and preservatives. You'll fill your refrigerator shortly (Step 2) with healthy, natural foods.

FINDING SUPPORT

Sticking to your diet in the beginning can prove difficult when close friends and family aren't eating the same as you. Even worse, they are eating all the things you're trying not to eat. Every person is different, and you likely know who will support you and who will not. For those who support you, explain that you're avoiding carbs (and which foods include carbs) and request politely that they not offer you anything when you're eating together.

Telling the naysayers that you've quit eating grains and sugar will usually suffice. The terms keto-vegan and low-carb will usually spark a debate or argument with certain people because they've been told their whole lives to eat carbs and low-fat products. Try to avoid using those terms when explaining your diet goals. Avoid direct debates by recommending they read about the benefits of being in ketosis and the health benefits of eating a low-carb diet.

Step 2: Go Shopping

It's time to restock your pantry, refrigerator, and freezer with delicious, keto-friendly foods that will help you lose weight, become healthy, and feel great!

VEGGIES

You can eat all no starchy veggies, including broccoli, asparagus, mushrooms, cucumbers, lettuce, onions, peppers, tomatoes, garlic (in small quantities—each clove contains about 1 gram of carbs), Brussels sprouts, zucchini, eggplant, olives, zucchini, yellow squash, and cauliflower.

Avoid all types of potatoes, yams and sweet potatoes, corn, and legumes like beans, lentils, and peas.

SWEETENERS …

The sweeteners may sound strange if you haven't heard of them before. They both come from natural sources and are safe to use in any quantity. Stevia is naturally obtained from the leaves of a plant by name Stevia rebaudiana. Stevia has zero calories and contains some beneficial micronutrients like magnesium, potassium, and zinc. It's readily available in liquid or powder form online and in most supermarkets. It's much sweeter than sugar, so containers are usually very small—you won't need nearly as much. Erythritol is a sugar alcohol that is low in calories, about 70 percent as sweet as sugar, and can be found naturally in some fruits and vegetables. Sugar alcohols are indigestible by the human body, so erythritol cannot raise your blood sugar or insulin levels. Several studies have proven it to be safe. Sugar alcohols can sometimes cause temporary digestive discomfort, but out of the few available sugar alcohols like xylitol, maltitol, and sorbitol, erythritol is considered to be the most forgiving and best for everyday use.

FRUITS

You can eat a small amount of berries every day, such as strawberries, raspberries, blackberries, and blueberries. Lemon and lime juices are great for adding flavor to your meals. Avocados are also low in carbs and full of healthy fat. Avoid other fruits, as they're loaded with sugar. A single banana can contain around 25 grams of net carbs.

DAIRY ALTERNATIVES

Although not technically dairy, unsweetened almond and coconut milks are great alternatives for keto-vegan diets as well. Avoid milk and skim milk, as well as sweetened yogurt, as it contains a lot of sugar. Avoid any flavored, low-fat, or fat-free dairy products.

FATS AND OILS

Avocado oil, olive oil, butter, lard, and bacon fat are great for cooking and consuming. Avocado oil has a high smoke point (it does not burn or smoke until it reaches 520°F), which is ideal for searing meats and frying in a wok. Make sure to avoid oils labeled "blend"; they commonly contain small amounts of the healthy oil and large amounts of unhealthy oils.

Step 3: Set Up Your Kitchen

Preparing delicious recipes is one of the best parts of the keto-vegan diet, and it's quite easy if you have the right tools. The following tools will make cooking simpler and faster. Each one is worth investing in, especially for the busy cook.

FOOD SCALE

When you're trying to hit your caloric and macronutrient goals, a kitchen food scale is a necessary appliance. You can measure any solid or liquid food, and get the perfect amount every time. Used in combination with an app like MyFitnessPal, you'll have all the data you need to hit your goals sooner. Food scales can be found online for $10 to $20.

FOOD PROCESSOR

Food processors are critical to your arsenal. They are ideal for blending certain foods or processing foods together into sauces and shakes. Blenders don't cut it, powerwise, for many foods, especially tough vegetables like cauliflower. One great food processor/blender is NutriBullet. The containers you blend in come with lids or drink spouts so you can take them to go or use them as storage. They're also easy to clean, making the whole system extremely convenient. They typically sell for about $80 online.

SPIRALIZER

Spiralizers make vegetables into noodles or ribbons within seconds. They make cooking a lot faster and easier—

noodles have much more surface area and take a fraction of the time to cook. For example, a spiralizer turns a zucchini into noodles, and with some Alfredo or marinara sauce, you can't tell you aren't eating noodles. Spiralizers cost around $30 and can be found in large retail stores and online.

ELECTRIC HAND MIXER

If you've ever had to beat an egg white by hand until you get stiff peaks, then you know just how difficult it is. Electric hand mixers save your arm muscles and massive amounts of time, especially when mixing heavy ingredients. You can find a decent one online for $10 to $20.

CAST IRON PANS

They've been used for centuries and were one of the first modern cooking devices. Cast iron skillets don't wear out and are healthier to use (no chemical treatment of any kind), retain heat very well, and can be moved between the stove and oven. They are simple to clean up—just wash them out with a scrub sponge without soap, dry them off, and then rub them with cooking oil. This prevents rust and encourages the

buildup of "seasoning," a natural nonstick surface. Many cast iron pans come pre-seasoned, and this method preserves the coating. You can find them in many retail stores and online for $10 to $80, depending on the brand and size; Lodge is a popular brand, still made in the United States.

KNIFE SHARPENING STONE

Most of prep time is spent on cutting. You'll see your cutting speed skyrocket with a sharp knife set. It's also a pleasure to use sharp knives. Aim to sharpen your knives every week or so to keep them in good shape (professional chefs sharpen their knives before every use). Sharpening stones cost under $10 and can be ordered online.

NICE-TO-HAVE EQUIPMENT

The kitchen section of any store can be a wonderland. There are so many intriguing gadgets. It's also nice (although not necessary) to have these other tools on hand if you can't resist the lure:

INSTANT COOKING THERMOMETER

Cooking steak and chicken is much easier when you can easily prod the meat and find out whether it's at the level of doneness that you're shooting for. These can usually be found for $10 to $20 in most retail stores or online.

MEASURING SPOON SET

Get the right amount of an ingredient quickly. These sets can go from $5 to $10 in any supermarket, store, or online.

TONGS

Tongs reduce splatter when working quickly (compared to using a fork or spatula to flip something in a hot pan). It's best to get tongs with nylon heads so you don't scratch any of your pots or pans. You can get a pair online or in retail stores for $10 to $15.

Step 4: Meal Plan

Using meal plans in the beginning of your diet greatly increases your chances of success. The meal plans in part 2 of this book include meals for every part of the day, premade shopping lists, and macronutrient and calorie counts for each meal. They even account for leftovers. This will make starting out much easier and more enjoyable!

Meal plans work well because they give you goals and direction. If you know what you need to make next without thinking about it, you're less likely to give up, change your mind, and order food from your favorite takeout spot. Also, since you know what's coming next, you can look forward to it throughout the day and week.

Pay attention to the ingredients listed on the packaged products you buy. The best products have just a few ingredients with recognizable names, meaning they're made with fewer additives and preservatives.

After using the meal plans for a few weeks, you set your body up to have the right expectations for how much food you'll provide it and what type of food it will get (high in fat and protein and low in carbs). Even if you don't continue to use meal plans, you'll be familiar enough with the diet to know what you should be eating and how much.

Step 5: Exercise

As you start your diet and the pounds fall off, think about how to lose more weight or get healthier to feel even better.

This is a great time to become more active through exercise.

Increase the amount you exercise relative to what you do now. If you don't exercise at all, start taking short walks or slow jogs, or a combination of both, for 15 minutes every other day. If you already go to the gym or lift weights, add an extra exercise or start doing cardio. It doesn't matter what level you're at, try to do a little more than you're doing now. That's all it takes to become healthier. Exercise is incremental, and every increment is a boost to weight loss and feeling better.

If you have the time, try taking a class or doing an activity that involves moving, like a step class or dancing, or start playing a sport like basketball. It doesn't have to be competitive, nor do you need to be good or have any previous experience. Such activities are an easy way to get on your feet, and you can learn a new skill in the process.

Staying fit through regular physical activity has been proven to reduce blood pressure and cholesterol levels as well as reduce risk for various heart diseases and type 2 diabetes. In combination with the keto diet, your health will improve dramatically, and so will your energy levels.

Any exercise, even if it's 15 minutes a week, is better than no exercise. Don't worry about how much you do in the beginning. Just start doing something and you'll build from there naturally.

EASY EXERCISE SEQUENCES

Here are a few easy exercise sequences if you're just starting out. Once every other day is enough in the beginning. If possible, try doing these with a friend or significant other for support and accountability. If you can't do some of them, that's absolutely all right! Simply focus on the ones you can do.

CARDIOVASCULAR ACTIVITY

Any aerobic activity, like walking, running, or bicycling, for 15 to 30 minutes, twice a week or more.

STRENGTH CONDITIONING

One set of exercises (for at least 10 repetitions, or it's too easy) targeting each of the major muscle groups: chest, shoulders, back, abs, and legs.

- Push-ups or assisted push-ups
- Pull-ups or chin-ups
- Crunches
- Squats

PART TWO

THE 7 DAYS MEAL PLAN AND RECIPES

CHAPTER 4

THE 7 DAYS MEAL PLAN

Here comes the long awaited 7 Day Keto-vegan Diet Plan! The caloric count of each day in this meal plan is set at 1600-1750 calories. However, if there is need for an increment, you can add more oils by lightly drizzling them over your meal or you can as well try adding one tablespoon of coconut oil to your coffee.

	MONDAY	TUESDAY	WEDNESDAY	THURSDAY	FRIDAY	SATURDAY	SUNDAY
BREAK FAST	Blackberry Coconut Breakfast Bowl	Blackberry Coconut Breakfast Bowl	Chocolate Raspberry Chia Pudding Shots	Curry Tofu Scramble with Avocado	Chocolate Raspberry Chia Pudding Shots	Curry Tofu Scramble with Avocado	Curry Tofu Scramble with Avocado
LUNCH	Chia Flaxseed crackers with Guacamole	Chia Flaxseed crackers with Guacamole	Garlic Brocolli on Cauliflower Rice	Garlic Brocolli on Cauliflower Rice	Asian Sesame Tofu Salad	Asian Sesame Tofu Salad	Asian Sesame Tofu Salad

DINNER	Almond Coconut Curry on Veges	Almond Coconut Curry on Veges	Tofu Spinach Curry (Saag Paneer)	Tofu Spinach Curry (Saag Paneer)	Tofu Spinach Curry (Saag Paneer)	Spinach, Avocado and Pumpkin Seed Salad	Spinach, Avocado and Pumpkin Seed Salad
DAILY SNACKS	1 1/2 oz almonds Mocha Protein Shake (No coconut oil)	1 1/2 oz almonds Vanilla Protein Shake (No coconut oil)	1 1/2 oz almonds Chocolate Protein Shake (1/8 cup coconut oil)	1/2 oz almonds Mocha Protein Shake (1/8 cup coconut oil)	1 1/2 oz almonds Vanilla Protein Shake (1/8 cup coconut oil)	Chocolate Protein Shake (1/8 cup coconut oil)	Mocha Protein Shake (1/8 cup coconut oil)
DESSERTS	Pumpkin Spice Fat Bombs	Pumpkin Spice Fat Bombs	Blueberry Fat Bombs	Spiced-Chocolate Fat Bombs	Chocolate-Coconut Treats	Almond Butter Fudge	Peanut Butter Mousse
TOTAL CALORIES	Calories (kcal): 1636 Fats(g): 130 Protein(g): 71 Net Carbs(g): 29.5	Calories (kcal): 1626 Fats(g): 130 Protein(g): 71 Net Carbs(g): 29.5	Calories (kcal): 1652 Fats(g): 137 Protein(g): 68 Net Carbs(g): 28.5	Calories (kcal): 1710 Fats(g): 142 Protein(g): 72 Net Carbs(g): 29.5	Calories (kcal): 1725 Fats(g): 140 Protein(g): 76 Net Carbs(g): 29.5	Calories (kcal): 1611 Fats(g): 132 Protein(g): 67 Net Carbs(g): 25.0	Calories (kcal): 1611 Fats(g): 132 Protein(g): 67 Net Carbs(g): 25.0

Planning Ahead:

Once your kitchen is organized for cooking, the next step is to plan an approximate weekly keto-vegan menu. Do this by writing out what meals you would like to cook for the next week. Do these BEFORE you do your grocery shopping. To make life a little easier on your busy nights, aim to cook meals that are fast to assemble. Plan one night where you can cook a double quantity of your recipe so you can reheat the leftovers for another night. On the weekend, try making two dishes and refrigerated one. Then give yourself a night off during the weekend.

Once you've written down this meal plan this way, create a shopping list to match it. Check your fridge or freezer and pantry to see which ingredients you already have. Go for grocery shopping after you have had a meal so you are not tempted to purchase a meal not on your list.

Keep your meal plan on the fridge or any other conspicuous place in the kitchen. When you arrive tired and hungry at the end of the day you will be really pleased to see the hard work of deciding "what's for dinner" is done. You will also discover you start to prepare dinner on auto-pilot mode.

ADDITIONAL TIPS

- **Aim for 1200-1500 calories per day, as a minimum intake to ensure you get all the nutrients you need form food to keep you healthy while you are losing weight.**

- **The ideal rate of weight loss is ½ to 1 kilogram of body weight per day.**
- **You may lose weight faster in the first few weeks due to changes in energy and water storage.**
- **If you lose weight faster than 1 kilo per week after the first few weeks, you can increase your average daily calorie intake.**

There are many facets to following a healthy lifestyle, but healthy eating should be at the top of the list. Finding time to plan meals is the greatest route to proper eating and healthy living and it starts with being able to know which foods to pick up from the grocery store and preparing the foods in such a way you will enjoy daily. These comes with some challenges to anyone who wants to plan and pattern meals in a way to feel energized and maintain or lose weight and feel energized as nothing good comes easy.. Many of us have full time jobs with aging parents to take care of; children and other responsibilities making us have busy schedules with little or no time for ourselves. The goal of this article is to outline some important meal planning challenges and point out the best ways to overcome them so you can eat right and live healthy.

Here is the most common meal planning challenges and their solutions or means to overcome them

1.   Healthy meals take much time to prepare
Solution:
Utilize precut vegetables and other healthy convenient

foods. Search for crisp onions, celery, carrots, chime peppers, broccoli, cauliflower, and mushrooms sold in the deliver path. Likewise use pre-marinated lean meats, rotisserie-cooked chicken bosoms, quartered marinated artichokes, preminced garlic and ginger, and canned beans, canned fish, and shredded reduced-fat cheddar to spare prep time.

2.   The kids usually have their separate meals and can hardly fit into the plan.

Solution:

Prepare 1 diet yet season it in 2 diverse ways. For example, on pasta night, make a striking tasting sauce for the grown-ups, but warm up bumped spaghetti sauce for the children. When making meals, partition the blend fifty-fifty, enhance every half in a different way, at that point fill the two sides of the meal dish and stamp them with toothpicks so you'll know which will be which.

3.   We often eat in restaurants and take some food home

        Solution

Reduce eating out or takeout suppers to once or at most two times every week. Rather than creamy or fried dishes, place order for dishes that are heated, cooked, barbecued, or steamed. Request that sauces and dressing be served by the side of your order. If your food does not contain enough vegetables, request an additional serving.

4.   Majority of our planned healthy meals don't really taste great.

Solution:

Tape a chart of herbs/flavors and their matching foods inside your pantry for simple reference. For instance, thyme runs well with chicken and mushrooms and rosemary with lean meat. Include seasoning with sun-dried tomatoes, hot pepper sauce, balsamic vinegar, and salsa or lemon juice for an additional lift.

PART THREE

PUTTING ALL RECIPES TOGETHER

Delicious Keto-Vegan Food Lists

BREAKFAST

1. Chocolate-Raspberry Chia Pudding Shots
2. Curry Tofu Scramble with Avocado
3. Blackberry Coconut Breakfast Bowl

DINNER

4. Almond Coconut Curry on Veges
5. Tofu Spinach Curry (Saag Paneer)
6. Spinach, Avocado and Pumpkin Seed Salad

LUNCH

7. Garlic Broccoli on Cauliflower Rice
8. Asian Sesame Tofu Salad
9. Chia Flaxseed Crackers with Guacamole

DAILY SNACKS

10. Keto Chocolate Protein Shake (Part 1)
11. Keto Chocolate Protein Shake (Part 2)
12. Keto Vanilla Protein Shake

DESSERTS

13. Pumpkin Spice Fat Bombs
14. Blueberry Fat Bombs
15. Spiced-Chocolate Fat Bombs
16. Chocolate-Coconut Treats
17. Almond Butter Fudge
18. Peanut Butter Mousse

BREAKFAST

CHOCOLATE-RASPBERRY CHIA PUDDING SHOTS

Dessert and breakfast, together once more! These Chocolate-Raspberry Chia pudding shots are relatively similar to enchantment. They're solid and sweet - the ideal mix. Celebrated for being a low carb thickening agent, these natural chia seeds make a remarkable pudding!

Course: Breakfast, Dessert;
Prep Time 1 hour;
Servings 2; Calories 240 kcal

INGREDIENTS:

- ¼ cup chia seeds

- 1/2 cup coconut milk

- 1/4 cup almond milk

- 1 tablespoon cacao powder

- 1 tablespoon Stevia

- 1/2 cup raspberries

INSTRUCTIONS:

1. In a container, bring together all the ingredients (with the exception of the raspberries) and shake vivaciously. Let sit for 2 minutes and after that fill four shot glasses.

2. Refrigerate for no less than 60 minutes (ideally across the night) until the point that blend thickens into pudding. Top with raspberries.

Recipe Notes:

This yield of this recipe is 4 shots. 1 serving is 2 shots.

Nutritional Information:

Calories: 241, Protein: 4g Fats: 20g, , Net Carbs: 4g

CURRY TOFU SCRAMBLE WITH AVOCADO

This tofu scramble is a fabulous low carb veggie lover approach to
begin the morning, with a lot of supplements and sufficient calories to
give you vitality for the day ahead.

Course: Breakfast;
Prep Time 5 minutes;
Total Time 20 minutes, Cook Time 13 minutes; Calories 380 kcal Servings 3

INGREDIENTS:

- **1 tbsp coconut oil**
- **2 tbsp olive oil**
- **300 g tofu (extra firm)**
- **1 tsp turmeric**
- **1 tbsp nutritional yeast**
- **1 tbsp curry powder**
- **1/2 cup zucchini (chopped)**
- **1 cup mushrooms (chopped)**
- **1 tomato (chopped)**
- **cilantro (optional)(to garnish)**
- **300-gram avocado**

INSTRUCTIONS:

- The initial step is to dry the tofu so it ingests the flavor.
- Cut the tofu into 1 inch long strips, spread out the strips on a paper towel,
- put another paper towel to finish everything and after that a slashing board.
- Place something substantial over this, for example, a few books.
- Abandon it to sit for around 15 minutes.
- Add the coconut oil to the dish and disintegrate the tofu into the skillet with your hands.
- Cook for around 5 minutes, mixing every now and again.
- Include the turmeric, nourishing yeast and curry powder and 1 tbsp of the olive oil,
- blend and cook for a further 4 minutes.
- Add whatever remains of the olive oil, zucchini, mushroom and tomato and sear for a further 4 minutes blending much of the time.
- Serve with 1 little medium size avocado (roughly 100g) cut.

Recipe Notes:

This meal can be refrigerated for a few days.

Nutritional Information:

Calories: 381, Fats: 32g, Protein: 11g, Net Carbs: 8g

BLACKBERRY COCONUT BREAKFAST BOWL

This breakfast bowl is smooth and rich, and has the magnificent FLAVORS of blackberry and coconut. An extraordinary begin to the day. It's likewise super simple and snappy to get ready!

Course Breakfast;
Total Time 5 minutes; Prep Time 5 minutes; Calories 467 kcal ; Servings 2

INGREDIENTS:

. **1 cup blackberries**

. **1 cup coconut milk**

. **3 tbsp ground flaxseed**

. **1/4 cup water**

. **1 cup spinach**

. **1/4 cup coconut flakes**

. **2 tbsp chia seeds**

INSTRUCTIONS:

1. Mix the flaxseed with the water in a glass until the point that the water is assimilated (just needs around 10 seconds).
2. Pour a large portion of the blackberries (sparing some for trimming), coconut drain, spinach and the flaxseed blend into a blender and mix until smooth.
3. In a different sear the coconut drops for a moment or two on high warmth to toast them.
4. Pour the berry blend into two dishes and sprinkle the rest of the ground flaxseed on top alongside the chia seeds and coconut pieces. Appreciate promptly.

Recipe Notes:
You can store the blackberry blend in the ice chest and utilize it the following day in the event that you like. Note this formula makes two servings - the beneath dietary data is for one serving.

Nutritional Information:

Calories: 465, Fats: 43g, Protein: 8g, Net Carbs: 7g

LUNCH

ASIAN SESAME TOFU SALAD

This Asian Sesame Tofu Salad is delectable, flavorsome and truly keto! The tofu assimilates the flours rice vinegar, sesame and tamari, while the zucchini, cucumber and spinach serve to keep it feeling new. The pumpkin seeds additionally include a decent crunch.

Course Dinner, Lunch, Main Dish, Salad; Cuisine Japanese; Total Time 33 minutes; Prep Time 10 minutes; Cook Time 23 minutes; Calories 406 kcal Servings 3;

INGREDIENTS:

For the tofu:
For the salad:

- **400 g tofu (1 packet, extra firm)**

- **4 cups spinach**

- **4 tbsp olive oil**

- **1 zucchini (sliced into thin strips)**

- **2 tsp tamari**

- **1 cucumber (chopped into semi circles)**

- **1 1/2 tsp sesame oil**

- **1 tsp ginger (crushed)**

- **2 tbsp rice vinegar**

- **1/4 cup sesame seeds**

- **1/4 cup pumpkin seeds**

INSTRUCTIONS:

1.   Mix 3 tbsp olive oil and the majority of the tamari, sesame oil, ginger and rice vinegar together in a bowl.
2.   Cut the tofu into 1 inch long strips and put into a skillet on medium high warmth. Include 1/2 of the dressing to the container and coat the tofu. Sear for around 10-15 minutes, precisely blending the pieces around in oil at regular intervals with a spatula until the point when the tofu is brilliant dark colored. Include the sesame seeds and 1/4 of the dressing to the dish and broil with the tofu for 2-3 minutes.
3.   Add the zucchini and cucumber to the bowl with the rest of the 1/4 of the dressing. Mix precisely for around 5 minutes. Expel from the warmth.
4.   Heat a little griddle at medium, include 1 tbsp of olive oil and the pumpkin seeds. Sear for a couple of minutes until toasted.
5.   Serve the Asian tofu over crude spinach leaves, and best with toasted pumpkin seeds.

Recipe Notes:

Stir the tofu with the oil carefully so as not to break.

Nutritional Information:

Calories: 407, Fats: 34g, Protein: 14g, Net Carbs: 7g

GARLIC BROCCOLI ON CAULIFLOWER RICE

This meal is so basic and is a staple for us. The supplement thick broccoli and the light and completely cauliflower rice mix well with the kinds of garlic and oil.

Course Dinner, Lunch;

Prep Time 5 minutes; Cook Time 10 minutes;

Total Time 15 minutes;

Servings 2; Calories 323 kcal

INGREDIENTS:

For the Broccoli:

For the cauliflower rice:

- **1.5 cup broccoli (chopped into florets)**
- **1.5 cup Cauliflower (chopped into florets)**
- **3 tablespoons extra-virgin olive oil**
- **2 cloves garlic (crushed)**
- **1/2 cup pumpkin seeds**
- **1 tbsp lemon juice**
- **salt (to taste)**

INSTRUCTIONS:

1. Put the cauliflower florets into a sustenance processor and heartbeat a couple of times until the point when it transforms into minor rice measured granules. Set aside.

2. Place a dish on medium high warmth and pour in 1 tbsp of the olive oil, pounded garlic and pumpkin

seeds. Warmth for a couple of minutes to toast the pumpkin seeds and discharge the kind of the garlic.

3.	Add the broccoli to the dish and panfry for around 5 minutes.

4.	Add the lemon squeeze and salt and panfry for an additional 2 minutes.

5.	Serve on promptly with the crude cauliflower rice and sprinkle 1 tbsp of olive oil over the highest point of each serving.

Recipe Notes:

Don't hesitate to swap the broccoli out for other low carb vegetables. Now and then we'll cook 1/2 container mushrooms and 1/2 measure of zucchini with the supper instead of the asparagus. Eat an assortment of vegetables in your eating routine. Additionally be liberal with the garlic as it works as the essential flavor. In the event that you need to include/decrease the calories simply alter the additional olive oil. You can likewise swap out the pumpkin seeds for Hemp Seeds or another seed on the off chance that you like.

Nutritional Information:
Calories: 322, Fats: 30g, Protein: 7g, Net Carbs: 8g

CHIA FLAXSEED CRACKERS WITH GUACAMOLE

These Chia Flaxseed Crackers make for an extraordinary dinner or tidbit. They're simple, cook rapidly and can be put away for utilize later in the week. An extraordinary keto-veggie lover feast.

Course Dinner, Lunch;
Cook Time 2 hours 20 minutes; Prep Time 25 minutes;
Total Time 2 hours 45 minutes;
Servings 4; Calories 256 kcal

INGREDIENTS:

For the guacamole
> **For the crackers**

- **1 avocado**
- **35 g whole flaxseed**
- **1 small tomato (chopped into 1cm cubes)**
- **50 g ground flaxseed**
- **1 lime (juiced)**
- **40 g chia seeds**
- **1 garlic clove (small, crushed)**
- **1 tbsp tamari**
- **1 tbsp cilantro (chopped)**
- **1 pinch sea salt**
- **1 cup of water**

INSTRUCTIONS:

For the avocado:

1. Mix the majority of the fixings in a bowl utilizing a fork until the point that the coveted guacamole consistency is achieved.

FOR THE FLAX SEED CRACKERS:

1. Preheat the broiler to 140 degrees
2. Mix every one of the elements for the chia seed saltines in a bowl and let the blend thicken for 15 minutes.
3. Warm a broiler plate in the stove, expel the plate and line it with preparing paper. Press the blend onto the heating paper, spreading it equitably. Prepare for 1 hour 40 minutes or until fresh. You may need to alter the time contingent upon the broiler, yet it takes a reasonable while.
4. After 1 hour 40 minutes the wafer blend ought to be decent and firm. Presently flip the blend over, turn the broiler onto fan barbecue and leave in the stove for an additional 40 minutes to fresh up the underside. You can build the warmth here with the end goal to lessen the time required, however be mindful so as not to consume the blend.
5. Remove from the broiler and cut into 4 areas, with 2 saltines for every segment. Present with the guacamole and appreciate!

Recipe Notes:

You can store the saltines in a sealed shut compartment in the pantry and essentially place them in the broiler for a fast 5 minutes before serving. Additionally take note of the picture we utilized for this completed formula is a twofold serving. You can have a couple of servings relying upon your caloric prerequisites.

Nutritional Information (One serving):

Calories: 256, Fats: 19g, Protein: 7g, Net Carbs: 5g

DINNER

ALMOND COCONUT CURRY ON VEGES

This almond coconut curry is super speedy and simple and tastes extraordinary as well! It flaunts nutritious vegetables alongside solid fats and a decent calorie tally.

Course Dinner, Lunch; Cook
Time 15 minutes; Total Time 15 minutes;
Servings 4; Calories 439 kcal

INGREDIENTS:

For the veges
For the curry

- **1 tsp coconut oil**
- **400 ml coconut milk**
- **2 cups mushrooms**
- **125 g almond butter (100% ground almonds)**
- **4 cups spinach**
- **1 tbsp tomato paste**
- **2 cups brocolli (chopped into florets)**
- **1 tbsp curry powder**

INSTRUCTIONS:

For the curry mixture

1. Put the coconut drain, almond spread, tomato glue and curry powder in a blender. Mix for around 20 seconds or until smooth.

2. Add the curry blend to a pan on low-medium warmth and warmth for 10-15 minutes or until warmed through. Blend habitually to abstain from staying.

For the veges

1. Heat the coconut oil in a container on medium-high warmth and include the broccoli and mushrooms. Sear for around 3 minutes. Include the spinach and warmth for one more moment.

2. Serve the veges in a bowl with the curry blend poured over the best.

Recipe Notes:

You can make the almond margarine by granulating almonds in a sustenance processor.

The curry blend isolates whenever left to sit in the refrigerator for some time, so make certain to mix it completely before utilizing on the off chance that you have put away it in the ice chest.
Nutritional Information:

Calories: 438, Fats: 41g, Protein: 11g, Net Carbs: 9g

TOFU SPINACH CURRY (SAAG PANEER)

A delicious vegan keto take on an Indian classic, this curry is simple, bursting with flavor and full of nutrition.

Course Dinner, Lunch; Cuisine Indian; Prep Time 10 minutes; Cook Time 18 minutes; Total Time 28 minutes; Servings 3; Calories 419 kcal

INGREDIENTS:

For the Tofu
For the Spinach Curry

- **2 tbsp Coconut oil**
- **400 g frozen spinach (thawed)**
- **300 g tofu**
- **1 Tomato**
- **1/2 tsp cumin**
- **200 ml coconut cream**
- **1/2 tsp garam masala**
- **4 cloves garlic**
- **1/2 tsp cayenne pepper**
- **1 tbsp crushed ginger**
- **2 cloves garlic (crushed)**
- **1/4 tsp garam masala**
- **1/4 tsp salt**
- **A pinch of red pepper flakes**

INSTRUCTIONS:

1. Cut the tofu into 1 inch long strips. Lay down a cotton tea towel and place the tofu on top. Folder the tea towel over onto the tofu and press down to drain the moisture. Do this for a minute or two, rolling the tofu over once to get all the sides.

2. Heat 1 tbsp of coconut oil in a pan on medium high heat and add the tofu. Cook for 10 minutes or until golden brown stirring frequently.

3. In the mean time Add all of the ingredients for the spinach curry into a blender and puree until smooth.

4. Add the garlic to the pan with 1 tbsp of coconut oil and fry for 3 minutes. Add the spinach curry.

5. Cook for a further 5 minutes to let the flavors absorb. Serve immediately.

Nutritional Information:

Calories: 419, Fats: 35g, Protein: 15g, Net Carbs: 10g

SPINACH, AVOCADO AND PUMPKIN SEED SALAD

This refreshing salad is delicious, vegan and keto and full of healthy fats and nutrients. The avocado tastes great, provides some decent calories and is nice and creamy.

Course Dinner, Lunch, Salad; Prep Time 10 minutes; Servings 2; Calories 400 kcal

INGREDIENTS:

- 2 cups spinach

- 1 cucumber (diced)

- 1 avocado (ripe, diced)

- 1/2 cup pumpkin seeds

- cups cilantro (chopped)

- 1 tbsp lemon juice

- salt and pepper

- 2 tbsp olives (sliced)

- 2 tbsp olive oil

INSTRUCTIONS:

1. Put spinach, cucumber, avocado, olives and pumpkin seeds in a salad bowl and mix together.

2. Toss with cilantro, lemon juice, olive oil and salt and pepper to taste.

Recipe Notes

This recipe is best served the same day it's made. Although it can survive in the fridge for a day or two - it won't be as fresh!

Nutritional Information:

Calories: 400, Fats: 36g, Protein: 8g, Net Carbs: 6g

DAILY SNACKS

KETO CHOCOLATE PROTEIN SHAKE (PART 1)

Course Drinks; Total Time 5 minutes; Calories 200 kcal; Servings 1.

This keto-vegan beverage is a staple for a veggie lover keto diet.

There are 3 variations intended to give command over what number

of calories you're expending without expanding net carbs. You can include

no coconut oil, 1/8 glass coconut oil or 1/4 container coconut oil.

With 1/4 container coconut oil the smoothie gives 31g of protein

and 670 calories, a significant number of which originate from

medium chain triglycerides which are fats that are effortlessly

utilized by the body for vitality. Contingent upon your calorie

needs, you can change the measure of coconut oil in this beverage.

INGREDIENTS:

- 1 cup almond milk (unsweetened)
- 2 Scoops Chocolate Protein Powder
- A few ice cubes
- 1/8 - 1/4 cup coconut oil
- A few cubes coffee ice

INSTRUCTIONS:

1. Pour almond milk into a blender alongside 2 scoops of the protein powder and a couple of ice solid shapes.
2. If you are utilizing coconut oil, place it in a different glass container and microwave for 45 seconds or until melted.
3. Turn the blender on and mix for around 30 seconds.
4. Now while the blend is as yet mixing, gradually empty the coconut oil into the blend. It should take around 10 seconds to pour all the coconut oil. This is critical to permit the coconut oil to completely blend into the smoothie and abstain from bunching or other repulsive surface impacts.
5. Drinks straight away, or put in the ice chest for tomorrow!

Turn this into a mocha shake

To make this a mocha shake, just make some dark espresso before hand, to empty it into an ice shape plate and put in freezer. Include these ice cubes to get a decent espresso flavor. Utilize decaf if you need!

KETO CHOCOLATE PROTEIN SHAKE (PART 2)

Recipe Notes:

This smoothie is a staple in the diet. The nutritional information for the no coconut oil, 1/8 cup and 1/4 cup coconut oil variants have been included. Simply modify it according to your needs!

Nutritional Information:

Calories: 200, Fats: 5.5g, Protein: 31g, Net Carbs: 3g

Nutritional Information with 1/8 Cup Coconut Oil:

Calories: 425, Fats: 32.8g, Protein: 31g, Net Carbs: 3g

Nutritional Information with 1/4 Cup Coconut Oil:

Calories: 671, Fats: 61g, Protein: 30g, Net Carbs: 2g

KETO VANILLA PROTEIN SHAKE

This delicious keto-vegan vanilla protein shake offers some assortment to your day by day chocolate shake. Similarly as with the chocolate form there are variations with including 1/8 glass, 1/4 container or no coconut oil. One advantage this one has over the chocolate shake is its net carb tally of 2g rather than 3g.

The ingredients are precisely the equivalent as the chocolate/mocha protein shake, with the exception of you'll utilize the garden of life vanilla protein powder (sport.

Nutritional Information:

Calories: 191, Fats: 5.6g, Protein: 32g, Net Carbs: 1g

Nutritional Information with 1/8 Cup Coconut Oil:

Calories: 415, Fats: 32.8g, Protein: 31g, Net Carbs: 2g

Nutritional Information with 1/4 Cup Coconut Oil:

Calories: 661, Fats: 61g, Proteins: 30g, Net Carbs: 2g

DESERT

PUMPKIN SPICE FAT BOMBS

Makes 16 fat bombs / Prep time: 10 minutes, plus 1 hour chilling time

Pumpkin is a great decision for desserts, particularly those that additionally incorporate warm flavors reminiscent of holiday pumpkin pie. Like its vegetable partner, carrots, the brilliant orange tissue of pumpkin shows it is an excellent wellspring of beta-carotene. Pumpkin is additionally high in nutrients An and C and in addition potassium, making this pretty fixing ideal for flushing poisons from your body and battling tumor.

INGREDIENTS

½ cup butter, at room temperature

1/2 cup cream cheese, at room temperature

⅓ 1/3 cup pure pumpkin purée

3 tablespoons chopped almonds

4 drops liquid stevia

½ teaspoon ground cinnamon

¼ teaspoon ground nutmeg

PREPARATIONS

1. Line an 8 square inch container with parchment paper and put aside.
2. In a small bowl, whisk together the butter and cream cheese until very smooth.
3. Add the pumpkin purée and whisk until blended.
4. Stir in the almonds, stevia, cinnamon, and nutmeg.
5. Spoon the pumpkin mixture into the pan. Use a spatula or the back of a spoon to spread it evenly in the pan, then place it in the freezer for about 1 hour.
6. Cut into 16 pieces and store the fat bombs in a tightly sealed container in the freezer until ready to serve.

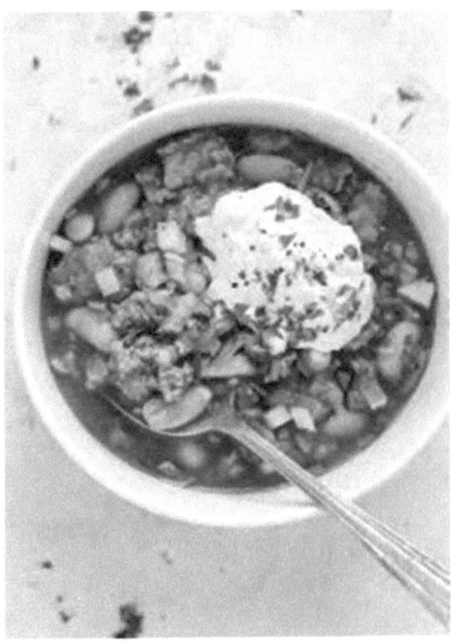

BLUEBERRY FAT BOMBS

Makes 12 fat bombs / Prep time: 10 minutes, plus 3 hours chilling time

The shade of these fat bombs is a particular blue, which you may discover startling in light of the fact that not very many nourishments are blue. Frozen unsweetened berries will work if fresh are not available or in season: Just thaw the frozen fruit first. On the off chance that your zone has wild blueberries, use these littler berries since they have an altogether more elevated amount of antioxidants against free radicals than grown blueberries.

INGREDIENTS

½ cup coconut oil, at room temperature

½ cup cream cheese, at room temperature

½ cup blueberries, mashed with a fork

6 drops liquid stevia

Pinch ground nutmeg

PREPARATIONS

1. Line a smaller scale biscuit tin with paper liners and put aside.

2. In a medium bowl, stir together the coconut oil and cream cheese until well blended.

3. Stir in the blueberries, stevia, and nutmeg until combined.

4. Divide the blueberry mixture into the muffin cups and place the tray in the freezer until set, about 3 hours.

5. Place the fat bombs in an airtight container and store in the freezer until you wish to eat them.

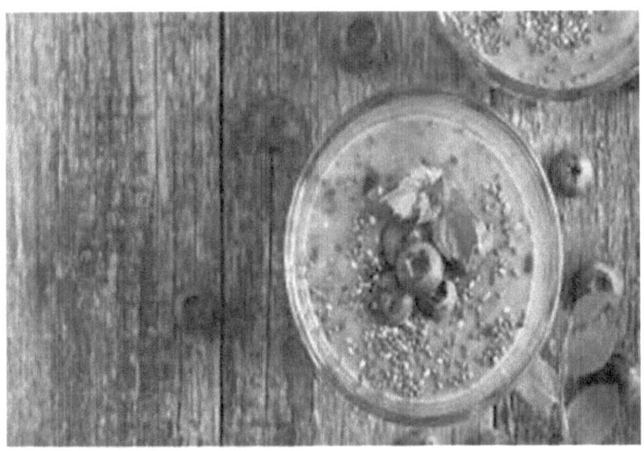

SPICED-CHOCOLATE FAT BOMBS

Makes 12 fat bombs / Prep time: 10 minutes, plus 15 minutes chilling time / Cook time: 4 minutes

Great quality cocoa powder is an adequate ingredient on the keto-vegan diet, which implies you can in any case appreciate a chocolate pastry and bite when you require a fix. Dull chocolate, for example, cocoa is high in manganese, magnesium, copper, iron, and fiber and also cancer prevention agents, which battle free radicals in the body. Dim chocolate has been found to enable lower to circulatory strain, diminish cholesterol, and enhance intellectual capacity.

INGREDIENTS

¾ cup coconut oil

¼ cup cocoa powder

¼ cup almond butter

⅛ teaspoon chili powder

3 drops liquid stevia

INSTRUCTIONS

Line a small scale biscuit tin with paper liners and put aside.

Put a little pan over low warmth and include the coconut oil, cocoa powder, almond spread, stew powder, and stevia. Warmth until the point when the coconut oil is dissolved, at that point race to mix.

Spoon the blend into the biscuit containers and place the tin in the fridge until the point when the bombs are firm, around 15 minutes.

Exchange the glasses to a hermetically sealed holder and store the fat bombs in the cooler until the point when you need to serve them.

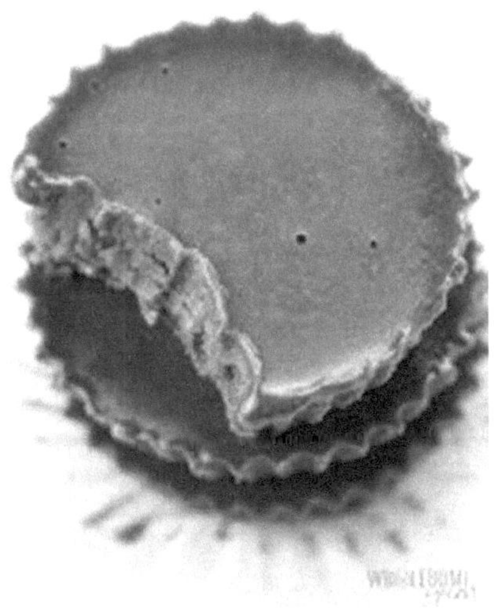

CHOCOLATE-COCONUT TREATS

Makes 16 treats / Prep time: 10 minutes, plus 30 minutes chilling time / Cook time: 3 minutes

Chocolate and coconut is a flawless combination often found in candy bars and many desserts. If you want a more elegant presentation, omit the coconut in step 3 and roll the semi hardened chocolate mixture into balls instead of spreading it in a pan. Then roll the balls in the shredded coconut and place the treats in the freezer to firm up completely.

INGREDIENTS

⅓ cup coconut oil

¼ cup unsweetened cocoa powder

4 drops liquid stevia Pinch sea salt

¼ cup shredded unsweetened coconut

PREPARATIONS

Line a 6-by-6-inch baking dish with parchment paper and set aside.

In a small saucepan over low heat, stir together the coconut oil, cocoa, stevia, and salt for about 3 minutes.

Stir in the coconut and press the mixture into the baking dish.

Place the baking dish in the refrigerator until the mixture is hard, about 30 minutes.

Cut into 16 pieces and store the treats in an airtight container in a cool place.

PREP TIP For a more finished look, you can spoon the hot mixture into candy molds instead of a baking dish. Pop the molds in the refrigerator for 30 minutes or until firm and pop the treats out into a cont

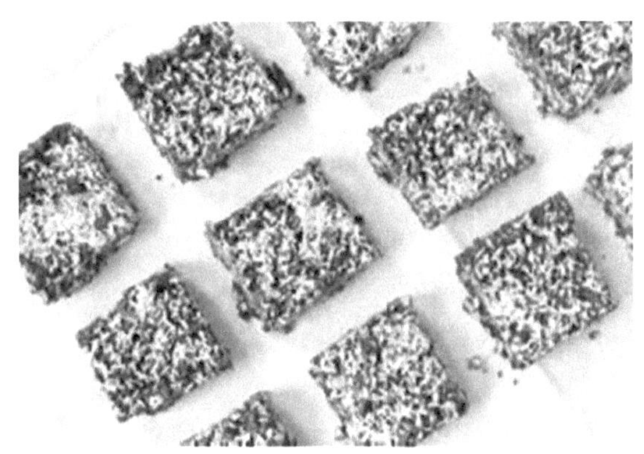

ALMOND BUTTER FUDGE

Makes 36 pieces / Prep time: 10 minutes, plus 2 hours chilling time

Fudge ought to be smooth and thick with no coarseness or graininess. Since you won't utilize granulated sugar for this treat, the odds of misunderstanding the surface are incredibly diminished. Almond spread is an excellent wellspring of protein, nutrient E, iron, manganese, and fiber. On the off chance that you are not a devotee of this nut margarine, nutty spread or cashew margarine would likewise be flavorful and make the equivalent enticing outcomes.

INGREDIENTS

1 cup coconut oil, at room temperature

1 cup almond butter

¼ Cup heavy cream

¼ Pinch sea salt

10 Drops liquid stevia

INSTRUCTIONS

1. Line a 6-by-6-inch baking dish with parchment paper and set aside.

2. In a medium bowl, whisk together the coconut oil, almond butter, heavy cream, stevia, and salt until very smooth.
3. Spoon the mixture into the baking dish and smooth the top with a spatula.
4. Place the dish in the refrigerator until the fudge is firm, about 2 hours.
5. Cut into 36 pieces and store the fudge in an airtight container in the freezer for up to 2 weeks.

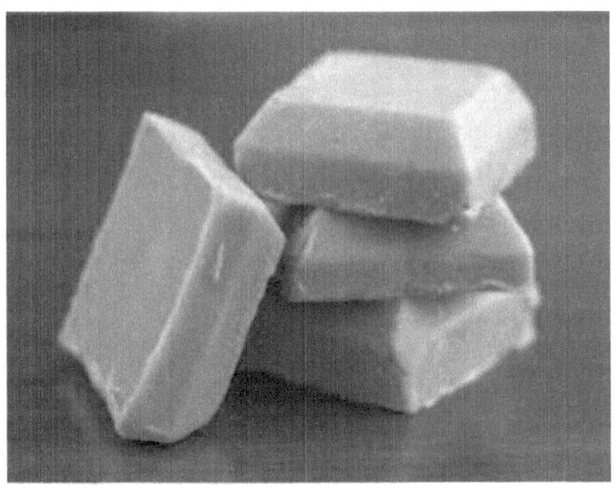

Serves 4 / Prep time: 10 minutes, plus 30 minutes chilling time

Peanut spread is dependably a convenient, delectable sandwich spread, however it is utilized in numerous kinds of dishes everywhere throughout the world, and is extremely sound. Eating nutty spread, even in this delectable sweet, can decrease your danger of malignancy and coronary illness, and help bring down cholesterol levels. Common nutty spread is high in unsaturated fats, protein, fiber, and folate.

INGREDIENTS

1 cup heavy (whipping) cream

¼ cup natural peanut butter

1 teaspoon alcohol-free pure vanilla extract

4 drops liquid stevia

INSTRUCTION

1. In a medium bowl, beat together the heavy cream, peanut butter, vanilla, and stevia until firm peaks form, about 5 minutes.

2. Spoon the mousse into 4 bowls and place in the

refrigerator to chill for 30 minutes.

3. Serve.

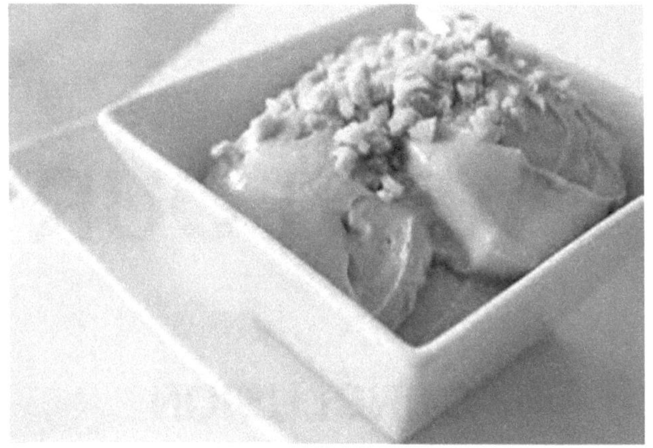

PART FOUR

CONCLUSION

HOUSEHOLD WEIGHTS AND MEASUREMENTS

Teaspoons, tablespoons and cups

- 1 metric teaspoon = 5ml/5g
- 1 metric table spoon = 20ml/20g
- 3 tablespoons = 1/4 cup
- 4 tablespoons = 1/3 cup

Oven Temperatures

OVEN TEMPERATURES	®C (CELCIUS)	®F (FAHRENHEIT)
VERY SLOW	120	250
SLOW	150	300
MODERATELY SLOW	160	325
MODERATE	180	350

MODERATELY HOT	**190**	**375**
HOT	**200**	**400**
VERY HOT	**220-250**	**450-500**

N.B. When using a fan-forced oven, decrease the oven temperature by 20 ®C.

ADVICE FOR EATING IN THE RESTAURANT

Getting rid of all culinary temptations is great for eating at home, but what happens when you go out to eat? Staying on a low-carb diet might seem difficult at first, but it can be easy with these few tips and a little bit of practice!

BREAKFAST

Skip the bagels, pancakes, Belgian waffles, French toast, or anything of the like. Opt for a side of sausage or ham. Skip the toast and hash browns.

LUNCH

Get a salad or garden salad. Use plenty of olive oil and salt (electrolytes). You'll feel great afterward and have plenty of energy to last you until dinner. Carbs are why people get sleepy after lunch. Don't be a victim!

DINNER

When ordering a burger, ask to have it wrapped in lettuce. If they're unable to do that, just ask for no bun. If they bring the bun, take the patty and anything else off the bun and put it to the side. Skip the ketchup as well—it's full of sugar. Try mayo, mustard, red pepper sauce, sriracha, or any other low-carb sauce.

At Italian restaurants, skip the pasta and pizza, and order the protein-based dinners. Make sure to request salad or any other low-carb alternatives instead of the usual high-carb sides. If all else fails, just eat the topping off of the pizza and avoid the crust.

With Mexican cuisine, try to get your food in a bowl instead of in a burrito wrap or tortilla. Don't get rice or beans; instead, get extra sour cream and guacamole.

SIDES

French fries, steak fries, mashed potatoes, baked potatoes, rice, beans, corn on the cob, banana bread, and any other high-carb sides can be replaced with salad, asparagus, broccoli, green beans, or other low-carb vegetables. Most restaurants have some sort of salad for you to choose from. Make sure to always ask and double-check with the waiter or staff.

DRINKS AND ALCOHOL

Instead of juice or soda, stick to water, tea, and coffee. Use heavy cream or half-and-half instead of milk.

In addition to fat, carbs, and protein, alcohol is also a macronutrient. It provides 7 calories per gram, the second most after fat, which provides 9 calories per gram. It is burned by the body before all the other macronutrients. If you drink too much alcohol, you will slow down your fat-burning process and impede your weight loss, if that is your goal.

If you're ordering alcohol, stay away from any cocktails, as they're all loaded with sugar. Dry or semidry wine has about 3 grams of carbs per glass, and lowcarb beers like Michelob Ultra and Modelo have 3 to 4 grams of carbs per bottle. All pure spirits like vodka, Cognac, brandy, bourbon, whisky, rum, tequila, and gin are zero carbs. As always, drink in moderation, stay safe, and enjoy!

RESOURCES

WEBSITES AND BLOGS

dietdoctor.com

Diet Doctor is a low-carb-focused site that provides articles and recipes as well as instructional videos and support.

ketodietapp.com

Keto Diet App is a keto-only blog and a great resource for science-backed articles and recipes. It also has an app for mobile devices which includes recipes, articles, meal planning, and progress tracking.

tasteaholics.com

Tasteaholics is a keto-centric website and resource which provides science-backed articles and recipes.

authoritynutrition.com/ketogenic-diet-101

Authority Nutrition is not keto-centric, but it provides many science-backed articles and is a great resource overall.

alldayidreamaboutfood.com

One of the oldest low-carb recipe blogs, with more recipes than any other low-carb blog.

reddit.com/r/keto

A large community with hundreds of thousands of users, who discuss progress, share cravings, and support each other.

BOOKS

Moore, Jimmy, and Eric Westman. *Keto Clarity: Your Definitive Guide to the Benefits of a Low-Carb, High-Fat Diet.* (2014)

Las Vegas, NV: Victory Belt Publishing. A great read and further look into the science behind the keto diet and benefits from eating that diet.

Givens, Sara. *Ketogenic Diet Mistakes: You Wish You Knew.* (2014) Amazon Books. If you hit a weight-loss plateau or are running into any issues, this book can help you break through and reach your goals.

APPS AND ONLINE TOOLS

Keto Macro Calculators:

keto-calculator.ankerl.com
The most detailed and complex.

ketogains.com/ketogains-calculator
A simple calculator with no charts and only numbers.

MyFitnessPal (app)
A diet and exercise journal which provides meal tracking, calorie and macronutrient tracking, automatic calculation of meal nutrition, exercise tracking and caloric spend, and much more.

Keto Vegan

Eat Right, Not Less

By:

Holly R.Evans

Copyright © 2019 by **Holly R.Evans**

About This Book

As many people get to know about keto diet, it is becoming increasingly clear that there is no single "right" approach to accomplish and maintain ketosis. Many popular voices in the keto space offer a perspective that differs from the traditional, more dogmatic approach to low-carb eating. It has been really cool to watch the popularity of this diet grow over the years and to see the different tips, strategies, and even products that members of the keto community think of.
Holly R.Evans

TABLE OF CONTENTS

INTRODUCTION

A ketogenic diet refers to one that is low in carbohydrates, which will allow the body to break down fat faster in order to metabolize ketones.
It's also the inclusion of real food and wholesome ingredients. Besides, a vegetarian binging on donuts, fries, and cheese is doing their health and environment a disservice as much as any other food junkie.

Are you anxious to lose some unwanted pounds and looking for something that can burn fat at maximum speed? Have you tried endless other diet plans but didn't work for more than a few weeks?
This book is mainly for you.

WAY TO ACHIEVE MAINTAIN KETOSIS

We will explore what you need to know about ketosis

KETOSIS – WHAT DOES IT MEAN?

In the simplest terms, it is a state achieved when fat burning is active. The body starts burning fat and its proteins, in exchange for energy. We can talk about the state of ketosis when the concentration of glucose is lesser than that of the level of ketone bodies in the blood. The ketogenic diet is a low carbohydrate diet.

FASTER FAT BURNING

The body of each of us has an unwanted fat. Thanks to ketosis it is easy to get rid of it because the body burns fat tissue. Eating carbohydrates, the body first consumes glycogen stores (energy reserve used for physical activity), then fat. It is, therefore, a much longer process. If you do not eat carbohydrates, there is no glucose in your blood, so you ask where the energy is being taken from? The body, instead of insulin, starts glucagon at the moment, which is what breaks down the fat tissue - as it can not use sugars because we did not provide them. Energy, in this case, arises from the burning of fat stores.

SMALLER APPETITE

Ketone bodies, formed by decomposition of fats, limit hunger. Often, despite the small portion, the meal is high in calories due to its fat content. By excluding carbohydrates from your diet, you limit insulin fluctuations and hunger pangs caused by them.

HOW TO START?

It is best to take small steps to avoid feeling unwell and stomach problems that can occur with a drastic change in diet and sudden carbohydrate trimming. Initially, you can start with consuming 25-30% carbohydrates, 40% protein 35% fat. Then, observing the effects, we reduce carbohydrates by 5% to obtain a supply of 50-80 g of carbs a day.

The best way to enter the state of ketosis is a large intake of fats with a small amount of protein, and you can also eat about 50 grams of carbohydrates a day.

WHAT FATS CAN YOU USE?

Diversifying sources of fat is essential. It can not be based, for example, only on animal fats. Eat also fatty fish, olive oil, coconut oil, avocado, nuts, seeds and seeds.

FREQUENT ALLEGATIONS

How to function since carbohydrates are the source of the fastest assimilable energy, and glucose, which is processed after the body consumes them, is energy for the brain.

It is thanks to the abundant supply of fat that the body can produce ketone bodies that provide energy and food also for the brain.

Let's go back to our ancestors who did not know cereals, fruits or vegetables. Their primary source of energy was fats.

Now the question is, what about carbohydrates? Eat or not eat?

Follow and listen to your body! Personally, as an athlete, I do not recommend completely giving up carbohydrates, especially to active people. I am the most like this when it comes to carbohydrate intake after training.

Remember that if the active person's diet is low in carbohydrates, symptoms such as irritability, tiredness, sleep disturbances, loss of joy of life, and frustrations may occur. This will mean that the adrenal glands that are depleted with low sugar levels excessively produce cortisol. There will be a problem with obtaining glucose and creating energy by eliminating carbohydrates. Exhaustion of the adrenal glands causes difficulty in the conversion of glycogen. Then the thyroid slows down, the body is still cold, there is no desire for sex, you do not know when you are full and when you do not, you have a sweet, disturbed sleep, stop menstruating, gain weight.

And you need 50 - 70 g of carbohydrates a day to maintain a relative balance. I'm not talking about overeating bread or cereals in general. Remember that carbohydrates are also found in vegetables - potatoes, sweet potatoes, root vegetables or pumpkin.

If your daily energy expenditure does not require a large supply of carbohydrates, put on protein-fat meals, especially in the morning. Carbohydrate eats for a second breakfast. My observations confirm: if you want to significantly reduce carbohydrates and not lose health, then you need to increase the amount of fat in the diet.
Fat along with the protein give a significant signal of satiety but on the condition that you eat slowly and thoroughly biting. Such meals have a smaller volume than carbohydrates, and sometimes we eat more than we should, to feel full.

In case you care about the increase in muscle mass, it even requires increasing the amount of coals in the diet.

NOT FOR EVERYONE!!!

The ketogenic diet is not the best option for people with liver, pancreas or kidney problems. Managing a greater burden due to the metabolism of ketones will be a problem.

WHOM IS KETOGENIC DIET REALLY GOOD FOR?

For people with autoimmune diseases, with diabetes, insulin-resistant. Also for some cancers, for problems with the intestines like FODMAPS, issues with the absorption of sugars and fibre.

An example of a one-day menu proposed by me:
This is an sample of a one-day meal for an athlete

On an empty stomach:
 Protein (e.g., immunocal)

Breakfast:
Quinoa with sour fruits such as pomegranate and raspberries

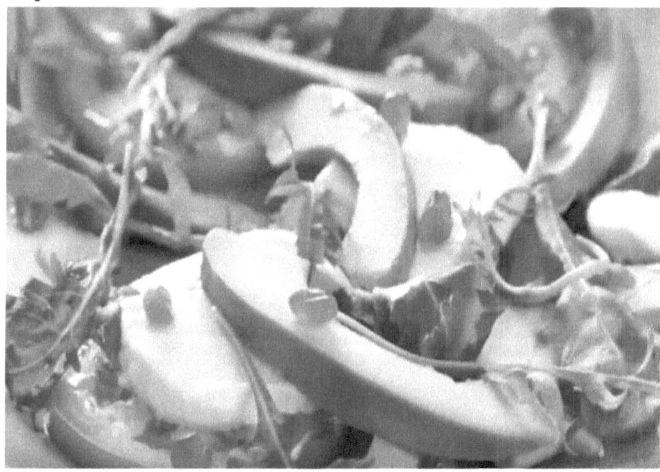

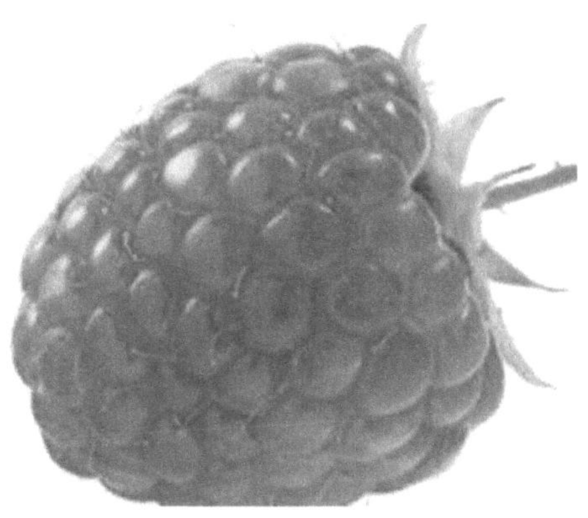

Training 10.00
Coconut water
Or mackerel paste with roasted peppers and olives

After workout
Cocktail with avocado banana and raw yolks and coconut water

Lunch
Tomatoes, zucchini, blanched spinach, beef steak

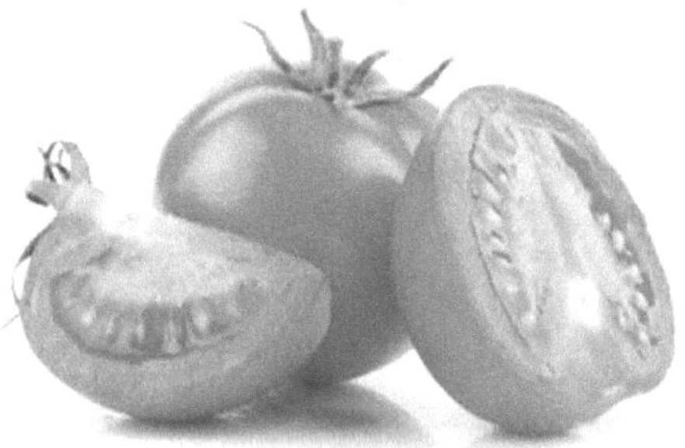

Tomatoes

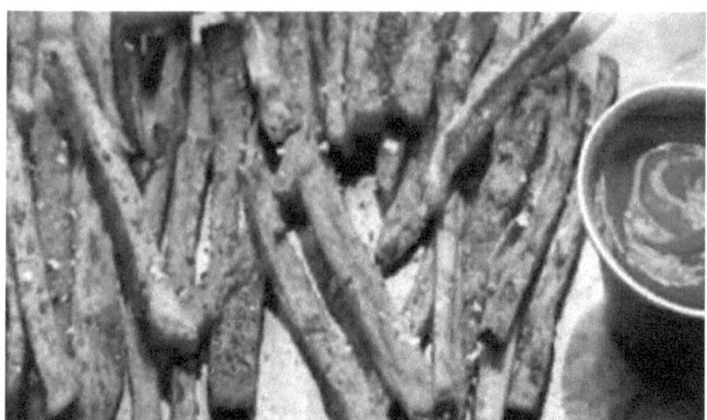

Zucchini

Dinner
Boiled vegetables (zucchini, broccoli, celery) with pork tenderloin stew in curry sauce on coconut milk and a leafy salad with a dressing made of balsamic vinegar
Tea, silage

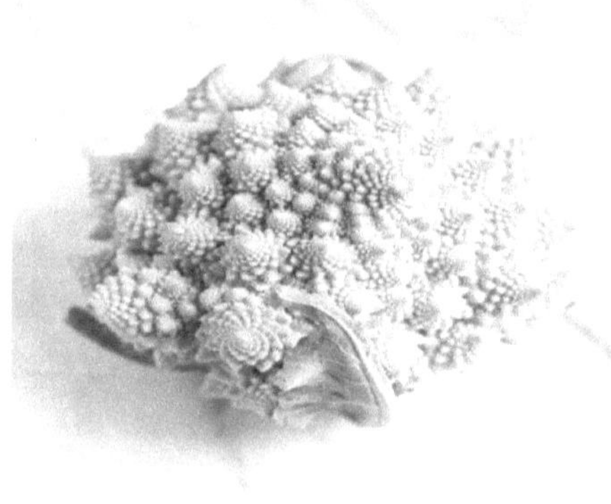

Broccoli

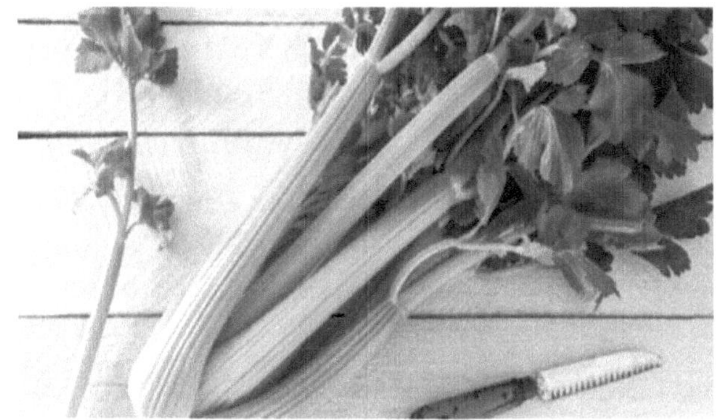

Celery

Supper

Steamed fish / baked in marinade with coconut milk, rosemary, sea salt, chilli

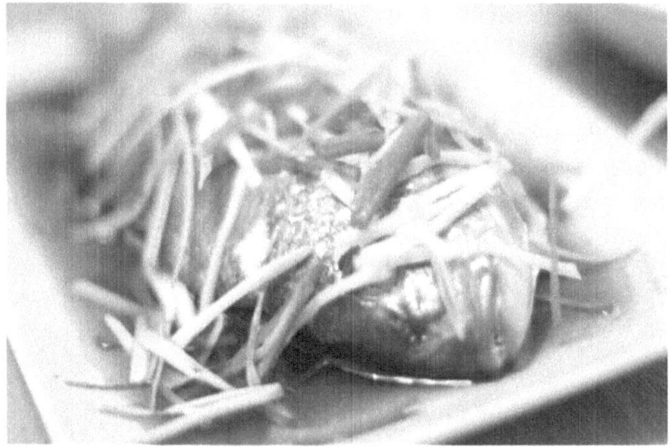

Steamed fish

CELEBRITIES ARE OBSESSED WITH THE KETOGENIC DIET

How celebrities like Meghan Markle, Gwyneth Paltrow, Ariana Grande, Kim Kardashian used Keto to transform their bodies and improve health

Meet 14 Celebrities Names Who Ditched Meat to Go Vegan or Vegetarian who are making us aspire to eat veg.

Meghan Markle

As rumour spread that Prince Harry has had his diet rebuild by Meghan Markle, however, is the Duchess of Sussex a vegetarian? When addressing Best Health in 2016 she expressed that when she was filming Suits, "I'm conscious of what I eat. I try to eat vegan during the week and after that have more flexibility with what I dive into at the ends of the week." So absolutely part time on the job, at that point!

Kim Kardashian

Kourtney's not by any means the only Kardashian who's been partaken in low-carb lifestyle. Kim has Joined the moving train, as well, and, as per report published in June 2016 in People, reportedly shed 60 pounds (lbs) after he gave birth to her child, Saint, while on the Atkins 40 diet. Atkins 40 is a variant of the Atkins diet intended for individuals with under 40 lbs to lose, and has been around since the 1970s. Atkins is basically the first keto diet and involves a very limited intake of carbs and high amount of fat. The fundamental different is that on the Atkins diet you'll gradually reintroduce carbs, so ketosis likely will only come into play during stage 1.

Gwyneth Paltrow

Paltrow has been known to dole out pretty wacky wellbeing advice through her health lifestyle brand Goop, like recommending body stickers to ease anxiety, as People reported in August 2017. According to a 2017 Bravo story, the actress and business mogul is a fan of the keto diet, which has a lot more research backing it up than some of her other claims. An report on Goop stated what the diet is all about and how to determine whether it's the correct one for you.

Ariana Grande

The newly engaged songstress has been veggie lover since 2013. As stated in an interview published in December 2014 in The Mirror, she did the switch in light of her love for creatures. "I love animals more than I love most people, not kidding," she said. She's agreed that eating out can be muddled yet says her typical move is to order what she knows is vegetarian — veggies, fruit, plates of mixed greens — and afterward fill up on other things once she's home. She has also spoken out about animal rights, as PETA noted, and against using animal products, according to MindBodyGreen.

Jessica Chastain

After having low energy levels, the Golden Globe nominee went vegan. Telling W Magazine about the experience, Chastain stated, "I simply had more energy than I've ever had in my whole life. I was just listening to what my body was telling me!"

Liam Hemsworth

The youngest Hemsworth sibling, Miley Cyrus fiance, and The Hunger Games star reportedly went on vegan in 2015. The impetus? "My own wellbeing and after all the information gathered concerning the mistreatment of animals, I couldn't keep on eating meat," he said in an interview published in November 2015 in Men's Journal. "The more I knew about, the harder and harder it was to do.." He's stated that eating in this manner has helped him both physically and mentally, he's encouraged his oldest sibling, Chris Hemsworth, to try it out, as well.

Serena Williams

Popular player to ever get a tennis racquet, Serena Williams went on an extremely strict diet after having her baby girl, Alexis Olympia. Talking at a Wimbledon press conference, Serena stated, "I was veggie lover, I didn't eat sugar!" The result of her change in diet didn't yield the results until the point that she ceased bosom sustaining, remarking, " I shed 10 pounds in seven days when I stopped. I simply continued dropping."

Will.I.AM

The Black Eyed Peas hit maker, Will.I.AM went Vegan in early 2018, stating via his Instagram post that he had joined the 'V.gang' Catchy.

Vinny Guadagnino

Guadagnino returned into the spotlight in 2018 with the reboot of MTV's hit reality television show Jersey Shore, called Jersey Shore Family Reunion. In the six years since the MTV show last aired, PopSugar reported in May 2018 that Guadagnino has embraced the keto diet and Create an Instagram profile with @ketoguido. He suggests eating bacon, butter, steak, fatty fish, plants, and exercising every week. As indicated by March 8, 2018, Instagram post, Guadagnino says his old method for eating had him 50 lbs heavier and looking 10 years older.

Madonna

As report stated by Thc Cut, the sixty year old superstar follows a super strict vegan macrobiotic diet which consists of cold pressed juices, fruits, vegetables and whole grains like quinoa.

Lea Michele

Formal Glee star Lea Michele used to treats her body like a temple, and turned vegan for the health advantages and also animal rights reasons. "It's tied in being good to your body and the planet. I'm a foodie, however I believe it's much more fun to discover things on the menu that are beneficial for me," she said. Lea was respected by PETA in 2010 for her philanthropy work with animals.

Jared Leto

The Oscar-winning actor Jared Leto and the rest of his 30 Seconds To Mars bandmates are generally strict vegetarians. "Indeed, here was a time when we used to sacrifice goats, but then we all became vegans, so we've been sacrificing tofu before the shows!" Good to know, Jared.

Adriana Lima

It take nothing to get the body of a Victoria's Secret angel. A low-carb diet and two-hour workouts each day. That's apparently what Lima did to prep for the Victoria's Secret Fashion Show a few years back, In an article publish from The Cut. Her diet was primarily made up of green veggies, protein, and protein shakes or cereal bars as snacks. Since then, it seems she's stuck to a keto diet, according to a story published in September 2017 in Harper's Bazaar.

Paul McCartney

When the beloved Beatle posed for an ad for PETA in 2008, he stated the moment he turned vegetarian, ABC News reported: "Few years back, I was fishing, and as I was reeling in the poor fish, I realized, 'I am killing him — all for the passing pleasure it brings me.' And something inside me clicked. I realized as I watched him fight for breath that his life was as important to him as mine is to me."

THE 10 IMPORTANT THINGS YOU SHOULD KNOW ABOUT THE KETO LIFESTYLE BEFORE YOU START

Want to eat less sugar, lose weight, and change your metabolism? The ketogenic or keto diet might work for you.

Here are things you should know before going on keto.

Not All Fat Is 'Good' Fat

Put simply, following the keto diet involves eating mostly high-fat foods. But this doesn't mean you can eat more fast food and dessert. Foods like avocados, eggs, and nuts count as optimal fat sources on this diet. Butter, cream, and other high-fat dairy and meat products do not.

It isn't a high-protein diet

On average, experts say protein should make up about 20% of your daily calorie intake. Recommendations don't change on keto. Instead, you're supposed to dedicate 75% of your calories from fat, 20% from protein, and only 5% from carbohydrates.

You're allowed to drink alcohol

Most alcoholic drinks are a low-carb dieter's worst enemy. But that doesn't mean you have to give up drinking entirely if you're on a keto diet.

Dry wines and light beers fall into the low- or no-carb category — you can have them as long as you drink responsibly. You won't lose weight if you spend all your calories on booze.

You shouldn't fast on the keto diet right away

When you first start the keto diet, your body won't quite know what's happening. It's best to make sure you're eating enough to properly adjust to the upcoming metabolic shift before making any more major changes.

This doesn't mean you can't incorporate methods like intermittent fasting into your diet once your body adjusts to ketosis. Just don't rush into it.

You don't have to stop exercising on keto

Whether this is good news to you or not — yes, a diet that discourages exercise IS too good to be true — you shouldn't avoid creating a workout schedule. Working out on this diet can be completely safe, as long as you keep them short, don't exert yourself too much, and switch things up from day to day.

You'll probably lose weight — at first

One dietitian tried the keto diet herself after more clients started asking about it. She said that even though effects like weight loss are certainly possible in the short-term, researchers aren't sure the same thing frequently happens in the long-term. Not many people stick with it that long.

Your gut may suffer

It's also difficult to include prebiotic foods such as onions, garlic, bananas and oats on a very low-carb, high-fat diet. "These foods encourage good growth of bacteria that support our intestinal health, which is tied to our overall health," says Julie Stefanski, a registered dietitian and spokesperson for the Academy of Nutrition and Dietetics. "But we don't know yet how the lack of fiber on a ketogenic diet impacts our microbiome or gastrointestinal health long-term."

You can't actually eat as much as you want

The keto diet forces you to cut back on many of the snack foods, desserts, and other high-carb options that could have made weight loss difficult for you in the past. But that doesn't mean you can eat infinite amounts of bacon and coconut oil. Consuming more calories, whether healthy or not, doesn't work.

Keto forces your body into a state of ketosis

When your body enters a state of ketosis, it burns fat as a primary energy source instead of carbohydrates. That's why you have to eat more fat and fewer carbs to reach this point. Ketosis is different from ketoacidosis — a life-threatening condition some people with diabetes develop.

Keto isn't the best weight loss diet for everyone

When Kirkpatrick tried the keto diet, she too experienced flu-like symptoms, which isn't an uncommon side effect when going on such a drastic diet. Chances are, you'll feel fatigued, you'll crave sugar obsessively, and you'll get a little "hangry." Headaches and nausea are also possible downsides.

Some dieters can't make it past these hurdles, and go back to their former eating habits.

THE BIGGEST MISTAKE PEOPLE MAKE WHILE BEING ON VEGAN KETO

It can be frustrating reading how others are successful with keto and you can't seem to be making any form of progress.

Fortunately, it's usually just a small thing preventing you from achieving your goals.

Below are some of the most common mistakes made by people that are starting a keto diet.

Too Much Protein

In a keto diet, you are going to need more fat than protein. Sometimes it seems as though some people forget this. They try to consume just as much protein as fat.

Doing this is going to slow down the weight loss process if that is your ultimate goal.

Having enough protein is really important for all of your muscles to function properly. However, consuming too much protein will cause your body to start turning some of it into glucose. The last thing you want to do when you're trying to eliminate sugars from your body is to have it make sugar from too much protein.

When you eat the right amount of protein, you'll be able to hold onto some of that protein instead of it being converted into glucose. This means your muscles will have some protein to use when it needs to.

It's not meant to be a permanent way of eating.

Although many people find weight loss success on the ketogenic diet, it's not a way of eating that's meant to be permanent. Due to its many restrictions, it can be difficult to do normal day-to-day things like go to drinks with friends or have dinner with family.

"Think of it as something you're going to do anywhere from eight to 12, to maybe 16 weeks," Mancinelli said. And continue to maintain a healthy, well-balanced diet after that.

Comparing Yourself to Others

Sometimes it's difficult, especially with the age we live in, to not compare yourself to others. However, when you're dieting, comparing yourself to others is one of the last things you need to do.

This is similar to the scale mistake talked about earlier. When you compare yourself to others, you're more than likely going to start stressing about the diet and have trouble focusing on it.

Stress has a major effect on your body whether you're dieting or not. You may not recognize how much it causes your body to change, but it makes a massive difference. If you're constantly stressed, you'll notice that your weight won't change as much as it probably should be.

On a keto diet, your body is going to react to it differently than the person next to you. That is why it is pointless to compare yourself to somebody else dieting. Everybody's body is different and will change different on any diet.

Focus on yourself when you're on a keto diet. If you aren't losing the weight right away, don't panic. The change is coming shortly. Keep your mind off the scale and stick with the diet and you won't be able to recognize yourself in a few short weeks.

Going About It By Yourself

Any diet is hard, but going about it by yourself will make the journey that much more difficult. Almost everything is easier when you have somebody to share it with.

When you have those moments of weakness (trust me, you'll have them no matter what) it'll be nice to have somebody there with you to keep you strong. If you and somebody else are embarking on the same journey, staying accountable for everything you do becomes easier.

Trying to hold yourself accountable can become difficult at times. When you have another person close to you to hold you accountable, staying with the diet becomes more of a goal instead of a daunting task which is always a plus.

Having somebody else with you on this journey allows you to share all of your struggles and successes with a person going through the same thing as you.

Not Enough Fats

When you start a keto diet, you will be consuming plenty of fats. However, there are many instances where not enough fats are consumed.
Growing up on a diet that was relatively low in fat and switching to a diet that is supposed to be high in fat could take some getting used to. You might feel as though you are eating too many fats, but more than likely, you're not.

This is why it is important to track your meals and see if you're meeting your daily macro goals.

It's important to just trust the process of the keto diet. Follow your macros even if it feels like you're eating more than you should.

You have your macros for a reason and sticking to that will give you the best chance at reaching your goals in a suitable time frame.

Looking For a Quick Fix

Some people think that going on a keto diet and cutting carbs is going to solve all of their weight problems fast and they can go back to their old lifestyles when it comes to food. This is false.

Starting a keto diet is something that you really shouldn't use if you want a Quick solution to your weight problems. Yes, you'll lose weight in the first few weeks, but if you go back to your old habits, the weight will come back in a hurry.

Ketogenic diets are lifestyle changes, not just changes for a few weeks. Switch to a different diet if you want to lose weight Quickly without changing your eating habits too much. Don't waste your time and money on a keto diet when it's going to last weeks and not years.

HOW TO LOSE 30LBS IN FEW WEEKS WITHOUT DOING HARMFUL EXERCISES

It is possible to lose 30 lbs. of bodyfat in few weeks by optimizing any of three factors: diet, or drug/supplement regimen. In this book, we'll explore ways to lose bodyfat without exercise.

Avoid "White" Carbohydrates

Avoid any carbohydrate that is — or can be — white. The following foods are thus prohibited, except for within 1.5 hours of finishing a resistance-training workout of at least 20 minutes in length: bread, rice, cereal, potatoes, pasta, and fried food with breading. If you avoid eating anything white, you'll be safe.

Eat The Same Few Meals Over And Over Again

The most successful dieters, regardless of whether their goal is muscle gain or fat loss, eat the same few meals over and over again. Mix and match, constructing each meal with one from each of the three following groups:

Proteins:

- Chicken breast or thigh
- Grass-fed organic beef
- Pork

Legumes:

- Lentils
- Black beans
- Pinto beans

Vegetables:

- Spinach
- Asparagus
- Peas

Mixed vegetables

Eat as much as you like of the above food items. Just remember: keep it simple. Pick three or four meals and repeat them. Almost all restaurants can give you a salad or vegetables in place of french fries or potatoes. Surprisingly, I have found Mexican food, swapping out rice for vegetables, to be one of the cuisines most conducive to the "slow carb" diet.

Most people who go on "low" carbohydrate diets complain of low energy and quit, not because such diets can't work, but because they consume insufficient calories. A 1/2 cup of rice is 300 calories, whereas a 1/2 cup of spinach is 15 calories! Vegetables are not calorically dense, so it is critical that you add legumes for caloric load.

Some athletes eat 6-8x per day to break up caloric load and avoid fat gain. I think this is ridiculously inconvenient. I eat 4x per day:

- 10 am – breakfast
- 1pm – lunch
- 5pm – smaller second lunch
- 7:30-9pm – sports training
- 10pm – dinner
- 12am – glass of wine and Discovery Channel before bed

Here are some of my meals that recur again and again:

Breakfast

Scrambled Eggology pourable egg whites with one whole egg, black beans, and microwaved mixed vegetables

Lunch

Grass-fed organic beef, pinto beans, mixed vegetables, and extra guacamole (Mexican restaurant)

Dinner

Grass-fed organic beef (from Trader Joe's), lentils, and mixed vegetables

Don't Drink Calories

Drink massive quantities of water and as much unsweetened iced tea, tea, diet sodas, coffee (without white cream), or other no-calorie/low-calorie beverages as you like. Do not drink milk, normal soft drinks, or fruit juice.

Take One Day Off Per Week

I recommend Saturdays as your "Dieters Gone Wild" day. Paradoxically, dramatically spiking caloric intake in this way once per week increases fat loss by ensuring that your metabolic rate (thyroid function, etc.) doesn't downregulate from extended caloric restriction. That's right: eating pure crap can help you lose fat.

A LIST OF KETO-FRIENDLY AND TASTY KETO-FRIENDLY RECIPES

Vegan recipes are like gold. Especially when they feature whole foods, and lots of plants. This type of cooking benefit your health and overall well-being in many important ways. No meat? No dairy? Don't sweat it. There are many other ingredients to get excited about when you're cooking and eating.

Here are some Keto Vegan Recipe you can start cooking in your home.

BREAKFAST

Keto Fat Bombs

These fat bombs are your best friend. Don't let the name scare you—these little balls are the perfect way to curb your hunger.

Yields: 8
Prep Time: 0 hours 5 mins
Total Time: 0 hours 25 mins

Ingredients

- 8 oz. cream cheese, softened to room temperature
- 1/2 c. keto-friendly peanut butter
- 1/4 c. coconut oil, plus 2 tbsp.
- 1/2 tsp. kosher salt
- 1 c. keto-friendly dark chocolate chips (such as Lily's)

Instructions

- Line a small baking sheet with parchment paper. In a medium bowl, combine cream cheese, peanut butter, ¼ c coconut oil, and salt. Using a hand mixer, beat mixture until fully combined, about 2 minutes. Place bowl in freezer to firm up slightly, 10 to 15 minutes.
- When peanut butter mixture has hardened, use a small cookie scoop or spoon to create golf ball

sized balls. Place in the refrigerator to harden, 5 minutes.

- Meanwhile, make chocolate drizzle: combine chocolate chips and remaining coconut oil in a microwave safe bowl and microwave in 30-second intervals until fully melted. Drizzle over peanut butter balls and place back in the refrigerator to harden, 5 minutes. Serve.
- To store, keep covered in refrigerator.

Nutrition Info

Per Serving: 84 calories; 8.4 g fat; 2.6 g carbohydrates; 2 g protein; 0 mg cholesterol; 0 mg sodium

Chocolate-Raspberry Chia Pudding Shots

Dessert and breakfast, together once more! These Chocolate-Raspberry Chia pudding shots are relatively similar to enchantment. They're solid and sweet - the ideal mix. Celebrated for being a low carb thickening agent, these natural chia seeds make a remarkable pudding!

Prep Time 1 hour;
Servings 2; Calories 240 kcal

Ingredients:

- ¼ cup chia seeds
- 1/2 cup coconut milk
- 1/4 cup almond milk
- 1 tablespoon cacao powder
- 1 tablespoon Stevia
- 1/2 cup raspberries

Instructions:

1. In a container, bring together all the ingredients (with the exception of the raspberries) and shake vivaciously. Let sit for 2 minutes and after that fill four shot glasses.

2. Refrigerate for no less than 60 minutes (ideally across the night) until the point that blend thickens into pudding. Top with raspberries.

Recipe Notes:

This yield of this recipe is 4 shots. 1 serving is 2 shots.

Nutritional Information:

Calories: 241, Protein: 4g Fats: 20g, Net Carbs

Curry Tofu Scramble With Avocado

This tofu scramble is a fabulous low carb veggie lover approach to begin the morning, with a lot of supplements and sufficient calories to give you vitality for the day ahead.

Prep Time 5 minutes;
Total Time 20 minutes, Cook Time 13 minutes; Calories 380 kcal Servings 3

Ingredients:

- 1 tbsp coconut oil
- 2 tbsp olive oil
- 300 g tofu (extra firm)
- 1 tsp turmeric
- 1 tbsp nutritional yeast
- 1 tbsp curry powder
- 1/2 cup zucchini (chopped)
- 1 cup mushrooms (chopped)
- 1 tomato (chopped)
- cilantro (optional)(to garnish)
- 300-gram avocado

Instructions:

- The initial step is to dry the tofu so it ingests the flavor.
- Cut the tofu into 1 inch long strips, spread out the strips on a paper towel,
- put another paper towel to finish everything and after that a slashing board.
- Place something substantial over this, for example, a few books.
- Abandon it to sit for around 15 minutes.
- Add the coconut oil to the dish and disintegrate the tofu into the skillet with your hands.
- Cook for around 5 minutes, mixing every now and again.
- Include the turmeric, nourishing yeast and curry powder and 1 tbsp of the olive oil,
- blend and cook for a further 4 minutes.
- Add whatever remains of the olive oil, zucchini, mushroom and tomato and sear for a further 4 minutes blending much of the time.
- Serve with 1 little medium size avocado (roughly 100g) cut.

Recipe Notes:

This meal can be refrigerated for a few days.

Nutritional Information:
Calories: 381, Fats: 32g, Protein: 11g, Net Carbs:

Curry Tofu Scramble with Avocado

This tofu scramble is a fabulous low carb veggie lover approach to begin the morning, with a lot of supplements and sufficient calories togive you vitality for the day ahead.

Prep Time 5 minutes;
Cook Time 13 minutes;
Total Time 20 minutes,
Calories 380 kcal
Servings 3

Ingredients:

- 1 tbsp coconut oil
- 2 tbsp olive oil
- 300 g tofu (extra firm)
- 1 tsp turmeric
- 1 tbsp nutritional yeast
- 1 tbsp curry powder
- 1/2 cup zucchini (chopped)
- 1 cup mushrooms (chopped)
- 1 tomato (chopped)
- cilantro (optional)(to garnish)
- 300-gram avocado

Instructions

- The initial step is to dry the tofu so it ingests the flavor.
- Cut the tofu into 1 inch long strips, spread out the strips on a paper towel,
- put another paper towel to finish everything and after that a slashing board.
- Place something substantial over this, for example, a few books.
- Abandon it to sit for around 15 minutes.
- Add the coconut oil to the dish and disintegrate the tofu into the skillet with your hands.
- Cook for around 5 minutes, mixing every now and again.
- Include the turmeric, nourishing yeast and curry powder and 1 tbsp of the olive oil,
- blend and cook for a further 4 minutes.
- Add whatever remains of the olive oil, zucchini, mushroom and tomato and sear for a further 4 minutes blending much of the time.
- Serve with 1 little medium size avocado (roughly 100g) cut.

Recipe Notes:

This meal can be refrigerated for a few days.

Nutritional Information:

Calories: 381, Fats: 32g, Protein: 11g, Net Carbs: 8g

Chocolate-Raspberry Chia Pudding Shots

Dessert and breakfast, together once more! These Chocolate-Raspberry Chia pudding shots are relatively similar to enchantment. They're solid and sweet - the ideal mix. Celebrated for being a low carb thickening agent, these natural chia seeds make a remarkable pudding!

Prep Time 1 hour;
Servings 2; Calories 240 kcal

Ingredients:

- ¼ cup chia seeds
- 1/2 cup coconut milk
- 1/4 cup almond milk
- 1 tablespoon cacao powder
- 1 tablespoon Stevia
- 1/2 cup raspberries

Instructions:

- In a container, bring together all the ingredients (with the exception of the raspberries) and shake vivaciously. Let sit for 2 minutes and after that fill four shot glasses.

- Refrigerate for no less than 60 minutes (ideally across the night) until the point that blend thickens into pudding. Top with raspberries.

Recipe Notes:

This yield of this recipe is 4 shots. 1 serving is 2 shots.

Nutritional Information:
Calories: 241, Protein: 4g Fats: 20g, , Net Carbs: 4g

Blackberry Coconut Breakfast Bowl

This breakfast bowl is smooth and rich, and has the magnificent FLAVORS of blackberry and coconut. An extraordinary begin to the day. It's likewise super simple and snappy to get ready!

Total Time 5 minutes;
Prep Time 5 minutes;
Calories 467 kcal;
Servings 2

Ingredients:

- 1 cup blackberries
- 1 cup coconut milk
- 3 tbsp ground flaxseed
- 1/4 cup water
- 1 cup spinach
- 1/4 cup coconut flakes
- 2 tbsp chia seeds

Instructions:

1. Mix the flaxseed with the water in a glass until the point that the water is assimilated (just needs around 10 seconds).
2. Pour a large portion of the blackberries (sparing some for trimming), coconut drain, spinach and the flaxseed blend into a blender and mix until smooth.

3. In a different sear the coconut drops for a moment or two on high warmth to toast them.
4. Pour the berry blend into two dishes and sprinkle the rest of the ground flaxseed on top alongside the chia seeds and coconut pieces. Appreciate promptly.

Recipe Notes:

You can store the blackberry blend in the ice chest and utilize it the following day in the event that you like. Note this formula makes two servings - the beneath dietary data is for one serving.

Nutritional Information:

Calories: 465, Fats: 43g, Protein: 8g, Net Carbs: 7g

LUNCH

Keto Chicken Enchilada Bowl

This Keto Chicken Enchilada Bowl is a low carb twist on a Mexican favorite!

Prep Time: 20 minutes
Cook Time: 30 minutes
Total Time: 50 minutes
Yield: 4 servings

Ingredients

- 2 tablespoons coconut oil (for searing chicken)
- 1 pound of boneless, skinless chicken thighs
- 3/4 cup red enchilada sauce (recipe from Low Carb Maven)
- 1/4 cup water
- 1/4 cup chopped onion
- 4 oz can diced green chiles

Toppings (feel free to customize)

- 1 whole avocado, diced
- 1 cup shredded cheese (I used mild cheddar)
- 1/4 cup chopped pickled jalapenos
- 1/2 cup sour cream
- 1 roma tomato, chopped

Optional: serve over plain cauliflower rice (or Mexican cauliflower rice) for a more complete meal!

Instructions

- In a pot or dutch oven over medium heat melt the coconut oil. Once hot, sear chicken thighs until lightly brown.

- Pour in enchilada sauce and water then add onion and green chiles. Reduce heat to a simmer and cover. Cook chicken for 17-25 minutes or until chicken is tender and fully cooked through to at least 165 degrees internal temperature.

- Carefully remove the chicken and place onto a work surface. Chop or shred chicken (your preference) then add it back into the pot. Let the chicken simmer uncovered for an additional 10 minutes to absorb flavor and allow the sauce to reduce a little.

- To Serve, top with avocado, cheese, jalapeno, sour cream, tomato, and any other desired toppings. Feel free to customize these to your preference. Serve alone or over cauliflower rice if desired just be sure to update your personal nutrition info as needed.

Nutrition Info
Calories: 568 Calories
Total Carbs: 10.41g
Fiber: 4.27g
Net Carbs: 6.14g
Protein: 38.38g
Fat: 40.21g

Almond Coconut Curry on Veges

This almond coconut curry is super speedy and simple and tastes extraordinary as well! It flaunts nutritious vegetables alongside solid fats and a decent calorie tally.

Time 15 minutes; Total Time 15 minutes;
Servings 4; Calories 439 kcal

Ingredients:

For the veges
For the curry

- 1 tsp coconut oil
- 400 ml coconut milk
- 2 cups mushrooms
- 125 g almond butter (100% ground almonds)
- 4 cups spinach
- 1 tbsp tomato paste
- 2 cups brocolli (chopped into florets)
- 1 tbsp curry powder

Instructions:

For the curry mixture

- Put the coconut drain, almond spread, tomato glue and curry powder in a blender. Mix for around 20 seconds or until smooth.

- Add the curry blend to a pan on low-medium warmth and warmth for 10-15 minutes or until warmed through. Blend habitually to abstain from staying.

For the veges

- Heat the coconut oil in a container on medium-high warmth and include the broccoli and mushrooms. Sear for around 3 minutes. Include the spinach and warmth for one more moment.

- Serve the veges in a bowl with the curry blend poured over the best.

Recipe Notes:

You can make the almond margarine by granulating almonds in a sustenance processor.

The curry blend isolates whenever left to sit in the refrigerator for some time, so make certain to mix it completely before utilizing on the off chance that you have put away it in the ice chest.

Nutritional Information:
Calories: 438, Fats: 41g, Protein: 11g, Net Carbs: 9g

Sesame Salmon w. Baby Bok Choy & Mushrooms

Ingredients

Main Dish

- 4 each 4-6 oz. salmon fillet
- 2 each portobello mushroom caps (or 8 oz. baby bella mushrooms)
- 4 each baby bok choy
- 1 tbsp toasted sesame seeds
- 1 ea green onion

Marinade

- 1 tbsp olive oil
- 1 tsp sesame oil
- 1 tbsp Coconut Aminos
- 1/2 inch Ginger grated (approx. 1 tsp.)
- 1/2 lemon juice
- 1/2 tsp Salt
- 1/2 tsp black pepper

Instructions

- Whisk together all of your marinade ingredients
- Drizzle half of the marinade on the salmon and turn to coat. Cover and refrigerate the salmon while it marinates for one hour.

- Preheat oven to 400.
- Prepare vegetables: Trim the rough ends from the bok choy and cut into halves. Slice the mushrooms into ½ inch pieces.
- Drizzle the remaining marinade over the vegetables and lay on a lined baking sheet.
- Place salmon, skin side down, on a lined baking sheet as well. Bake until salmon is cooked through, about 20 minutes.
- Top with sliced green onions and sesame seeds.

Caprese Tuna Salad Stuffed Tomatoes

Prep Time: 10 minutes
Yield: Serves 1
Serving Size: entire recipe
Calories per serving: 196
Fat per serving: 4.9g

Ingredients

- 1 medium tomato
- 1 (5oz) can tuna, very well drained
- 2 tsp balsamic vinegar
- 1 TBSP chopped mozzarella {1/4 oz.}
- 1 TBSP chopped fresh basil
- 1 TBSP chopped green onion

Instructions

- Cut the top 1/4-inch off the tomato. Use a spoon to scoop out the insides of the tomato. Set aside while you make the tuna salad.
- Stir together the drained tuna, balsamic vinegar, mozzarella, basil, and green onion. Put the tuna salad in the hollowed out tomato, and enjoy!
- Note: I prefer using fresh mozzarella but any mozzarella is good in here.

Loaded Chicken Salad

A delicious salad filled with plenty of vegetables and delicious grilled meat!

Prep Time 10 minutes
Cook Time 8 minutes
Total Time 18 minutes
Total Carbs 12.86g

Ingredients

- 1 boneless chicken breast (about 300g, with or without skin)
- 1 tbsp extra virgin olive oil
- 1/4 tsp Himalayan salt
- 1/4 tsp black pepper
- 1 avocado
- 100 g mozzarella balls
- 1 large tomato (any colour)
- 1 har artichoke hearts (my jar was 170g)
- 1/2 red onion
- 5 asparagus
- 20 leaves basil
- 4 cups baby spinach (200g used)

Dressing

- 2 tbsp extra virgin olive oil
- 1 1/2 tbsp balsamic vinegar

- 1 tsp dijon mustard
- 1 clove garlic
- pinch Himalayan salt
- pinch black pepper

Instructions

- Peel and dice the avocado. Slice the red onion. Dice the tomato. Pile the basil leaves together, roll them up and slice. Cut the stems off the asparagus and slice in half. Mince the garlic.
- Slice the chicken breast in half lengthwise. Sprinkle the 1/4 tsp of salt and pepper on each sides. Heat the 1 tbsp of olive oil in a cast iron skillet and place the chicken breasts in. Fry on each side, about 3 minutes each side, until they have a nice golden brown colour and cooked through. Add the asparagus beside the chicken breasts and cook a few minutes until soft and grilled. Take out the chicken and slice.
- In a small bowl, combine the minced garlic, olive oil, balsamic vinegar, dijon, and salt & pepper.
- Add the baby spinach to a large bowl or plate. Cover with the grilled chicken, avocado, mozzarella, tomatoes, artichoke, red onions, asparagus and basil leaves. Pour the dressing over and enjoy!

Notes

You can add 1 tbsp of honey to the salad dressing if you don't mind the extra carbs or want a sweeter dressing.

Nutrition Info

Calories 430 Calories from Fat 264
Saturated Fat 6.57g 33%
Total Carbohydrates 12.86g 4%
Dietary Fiber 6.12g 24%
Sugars 3.16g

DINNER

Keto Instant Pot Crack Chicken Recipe

Rich, creamy, and full of flavor, this Keto Instant Pot Crack Chicken Recipe is sure to be a favorite family dinner.

Cuisine: American
Prep time: 5 mins
Cook time: 20 mins
Total time: 25 mins
Serves: 8 servings (yields about 7 cups total)

Ingredients

- 2 slices bacon, chopped
- 2 lbs (910 g) boneless, skinless chicken breasts
- 2 (8 oz/227 g) blocks cream cheese
- ½ cup (120 ml) water
- 2 tablespoons apple cider vinegar
- 1 tablespoon dried chives
- 1½ teaspoons garlic powder
- 1½ teaspoons onion powder
- 1 teaspoon crushed red pepper flakes
- 1 teaspoon dried dill
- ¼ teaspoon salt
- ¼ teaspoon black pepper
- ½ cup (2 oz/57 g) shredded cheddar
- 1 scallion, green and white parts, thinly sliced

Instructions

- Turn pressure cooker on, press "Sauté", and wait 2 minutes for the pot to heat up. Add the chopped bacon and cook until crispy. Transfer to a plate and set aside. Press "Cancel" to stop sautéing.
- Add the chicken, cream cheese, water, vinegar, chives, garlic powder, onion powder, crushed red pepper flakes, dill, salt, and black pepper to the pot. Turn the pot on Manual, High Pressure for 15 minutes and then do a Quick release.
- Use tongs to transfer the chicken to a large plate, shred it with 2 forks, and return it back to the pot.
- Stir in the cheddar cheese.
- Top with the crispy bacon and scallion, and serve.

Notes

We've tested this recipe upwards of 10 times and have never had the burn warning come on; however, several readers have had the warning come on, so we want to give a tip. In step 1 of the Instructions above, after removing the bacon from the pot, we recommend adding a splash of water, and use a wooden spoon to scrape up any brown bits that have formed on the bottom to deglaze the pan. After that, continue on with step 1 and press "Cancel" to stop sauteing.

Nutrition Facts

Calories: 437 Fat: 27.6 Potassium: 390 Net Carbs: 4.3
Carbohydrates: 4.5 Sodium: 420 Fiber: .2 Protein: 41.2

Keto Chicken Enchilada Bowl

This Keto Chicken Enchilada Bowl is a low carb twist on a Mexican favorite! It's So easy to make, totally filling and ridiculously yummy!

Prep Time: 20 minutes
Cook Time: 30 minutes
Total Time: 50 minutes
Yield: 4 servings

Ingredients

- 2 tablespoons coconut oil (for searing chicken)
- 1 pound of boneless, skinless chicken thighs
- 3/4 cup red enchilada sauce (recipe from Low Carb Maven)
- 1/4 cup water
- 1/4 cup chopped onion
- 4 oz can diced green chiles

Toppings (feel free to customize)

- 1 whole avocado, diced
- 1 cup shredded cheese (I used mild cheddar)
- 1/4 cup chopped pickled jalapenos
- 1/2 cup sour cream
- 1 roma tomato, chopped

Optional: serve over plain cauliflower rice (or mexican cauliflower rice) for a more complete meal!

Instructions

- In a pot or dutch oven over medium heat melt the coconut oil. Once hot, sear chicken thighs until lightly brown.

- Pour in enchilada sauce and water then add onion and green chiles. Reduce heat to a simmer and cover. Cook chicken for 17-25 minutes or until chicken is tender and fully cooked through to at least 165 degrees internal temperature.

- Careully remove the chicken and place onto a work surface. Chop or shred chicken (your preference) then add it back into the pot. Let the chicken simmer uncovered for an additional 10 minutes to absorb flavor and allow the sauce to reduce a little.

- To Serve, top with avocado, cheese, jalapeno, sour cream, tomato, and any other desired toppings. Feel free to customize these to your preference. Serve alone or over cauliflower rice if desired just be sure to update your personal nutrition info as needed.

Nutrition Info

Calories: 568 Calories
Total Carbs: 10.41g
Fiber: 4.27g
Net Carbs: 6.14g
Protein: 38.38g
Fat: 40.21g

Crab Stuffed Mushrooms With Cream Cheese

An easy recipe for crab stuffed mushrooms with cream cheese. Low carb, keto, and gluten free.

Prep Time 15 minutes
Cook Time 30 minutes
Servings 4 servings
Calories 160 kcal

Ingredients

- 20 ounces cremini (baby bella) mushrooms (20-25 individual mushrooms)
- 2 tablespoons finely grated parmesan cheese
- 1 tablespoon chopped fresh parsley
- salt

Filling:

- 4 ounces cream cheese softened to room temperature
- 4 ounces crab meat finely chopped
- 5 cloves garlic minced
- 1 teaspoon dried oregano
- 1/2 teaspoon paprika
- 1/2 teaspoon black pepper
- 1/4 teaspoon salt

Instructions

- Preheat the oven to 400 F. Prepare a baking sheet lined with parchment paper.
- Snap stems from mushrooms, discarding the stems and placing the mushroom caps on the baking sheet 1 inch apart from each other. Season the mushroom caps with salt.
- In a large mixing bowl, combine all filling ingredients and stir until well-mixed without any lumps of cream cheese. Stuff the mushroom caps with the mixture. Evenly sprinkle parmesan cheese on top of the stuffed mushrooms.
- Bake at 400 F until the mushrooms are very tender and the stuffing is nicely browned on top, about 30 minutes. Top with parsley and serve while hot.

Nutrition Notes

This recipe yields 5 g net carbs per serving (5-6 stuffed mushrooms).

Nutrition Info

Calories 160
Total Carb 5.5g 2%
Dietary Fiber 0.5g 1%
Sugars 0g
Protein 9g

DESERT

Blueberry Fat Bombs

Makes 12 fat bombs / Prep time: 10 minutes, plus 3 hours chilling time

The shade of these fat bombs is a particular blue, which you may discover startling in light of the fact that not very many nourishments are blue. Frozen unsweetened berries will work if fresh are not available or in season: Just thaw the frozen fruit first. On the off chance that your zone has wild blueberries, use these little berries since they have an altogether more elevated amount of antioxidants against free radicals than grown blueberries.

Ingredients

- ½ cup coconut oil, at room temperature
- ½ cup cream cheese, at room temperature
- ½ cup blueberries, mashed with a fork
- 6 drops liquid stevia

Pinch ground nutmeg

Instructions

- Line a smaller scale biscuit tin with paper liners and put aside.
- In a medium bowl, stir together the coconut oil and cream cheese until well blended.
- Stir in the blueberries, stevia, and nutmeg until

combined.
- Divide the blueberry mixture into the muffin cups and place the tray in the freezer until set, about 3 hours.
- Place the fat bombs in an airtight container and store in the freezer until you wish to eat them.

Spiced-Chocolate Fat Bombs

Makes 12 fat bombs / Prep time: 10 minutes, plus 15 minutes chilling time / Cook time: 4 minutes

Great quality cocoa powder is an adequate ingredient on the keto-vegan diet, which implies you can, in any case, appreciate a chocolate pastry and bite when you require a fix. Dull chocolate, for example, cocoa is high in manganese, magnesium, copper, iron, and fiber and also cancer prevention agents, which battle free radicals in the body. Dim chocolate has been found to enable lower to circulatory strain, diminish cholesterol, and enhance intellectual capacity.

Ingredients

- ¾ cup coconut oil
- ¼ cup cocoa powder
- ¼ cup almond butter
- ⅛ teaspoon chili powder
- 3 drops liquid stevia

Instructions

- Line a small scale biscuit tin with paper liners and put aside.

- Put a little pan over low warmth and include the coconut oil, cocoa powder, almond spread, stew powder, and stevia. Warmth until the point when the coconut oil is dissolved, at that point race to mix.

- Spoon the blend into the biscuit containers and place the tin in the fridge until the point when the bombs are firm around 15 minutes.

- Exchange the glasses to a hermetically sealed holder and store the fat bombs in the cooler until the point when you need to serve them.

Chocolate-Coconut Treats

Makes 16 treats / Prep time: 10 minutes, plus 30 minutes chilling time / Cook time: 3 minutes

Chocolate and coconut is a flawless combination often found in candy bars and many desserts. If you want a more elegant presentation, omit the coconut in step 3 and roll the semi-hardened chocolate mixture into balls instead of spreading it in a pan. Then roll the balls in the shredded coconut and place the treats in the freezer to firm up completely.

Ingredients

- ⅓ cup coconut oil
- ¼ cup unsweetened cocoa powder
- 4 drops liquid stevia Pinch sea salt
- ¼ cup shredded unsweetened coconut

Instructions

- Line a 6-by-6-inch baking dish with parchment paper and set aside.

- In a small saucepan over low heat, stir together the coconut oil, cocoa, stevia, and salt for about 3 minutes.
- Stir in the coconut and press the mixture into the baking dish.
- Place the baking dish in the refrigerator until

the mixture is hard, about 30 minutes.

- Cut into 16 pieces and store the treats in an airtight container in a cool place.

PREP TIP For a more finished look, you can spoon the hot mixture into candy molds instead of a baking dish. Pop the molds in the refrigerator for 30 minutes or until firm and pop the treats out into a cont

Almond Butter Fudge

Makes 36 pieces / Prep time: 10 minutes, plus 2 hours chilling time

Fudge ought to be smooth and thick with no coarseness or graininess. Since you won't utilize granulated sugar for this treat, the odds of misunderstanding the surface are incredibly diminished. Almond spread is an excellent wellspring of protein, nutrient E, iron, manganese, and fiber. On the off chance that you are not a devotee of this nut margarine, nutty spread or cashew margarine would likewise be flavorful and make the equivalent enticing outcomes.

Ingredients

- 1 cup coconut oil, at room temperature
- 1 cup almond butter
- ¼ Cup heavy cream
- ¼ Pinch sea salt
- 10 Drops liquid stevia

Instructions

- Line a 6-by-6-inch baking dish with parchment paper and set aside.

- In a medium bowl, whisk together the coconut oil, almond butter, heavy cream, stevia, and salt until very smooth.

- Spoon the mixture into the baking dish and smooth the top with a spatula.
- Place the dish in the refrigerator until the fudge is firm, about 2 hours.

Cut into 36 pieces and store the fudge in an airtight container in the freezer for up to 2 weeks.

Peanut Butter Mousse

Serves 4 / Prep time: 10 minutes, plus 30 minutes chilling time

Peanut spread is dependably a convenient, delectable sandwich spread, however, it is utilized in numerous kinds of dishes everywhere throughout the world, and is extremely sound. Eating nutty spread, even in this delectable sweet, can decrease your danger of malignancy and coronary illness, and help bring down cholesterol levels. Common nutty spread is high in unsaturated fats, protein, fiber, and folate.

Ingredients

- 1 cup heavy (whipping) cream
- ¼ cup natural peanut butter
- 1 teaspoon alcohol-free pure vanilla extract
- 4 drops liquid stevia

Instructions

- In a medium bowl, beat together the heavy cream, peanut butter, vanilla, and stevia until firm peaks form, about 5 minutes.

- Spoon the mousse into 4 bowls and place in the refrigerator to chill for 30 minutes.

- Serve.

OTHER KETO VEGAN RECIPE

Cauliflower Pizza Crust

Prep Time 10 minutes
Cook Time 1 hour 10 minutes
Total Time 1 hour 20 minutes
Servings 6 1/2 " crusts
Calories 340 kcal

Ingredients

- 6 cups cauliflower florets 1 head
- 1 cup ground flax seeds
- 2 teaspoons basil
- 2 teaspoons oregano
- 1/2 cup nutritional yeast
- 2 tablespoons olive oil + more for oiling baking sheet
- 1 teaspoon onion powder
- 1 teaspoon garlic powder
- salt and pepper

Instructions

- Preheat oven to 400°.
- Steam cauliflower 10-15 minutes until tender. Let cool.
- In a cheesecloth or towel, squeeze out as much water as you can*. This will shrink the amount of cauliflower to about 3 cups.
- Put cauliflower and the rest of ingredients into a food processor and mix thoroughly.

- Spread 1/4 of ingredients (depending upon the size of your pizza) onto an oiled baking sheet or parchment paper. With slightly wet hands (dough is sticky), spread out the dough to about 1/4" thick, pressing the cauliflower in firmly.
- Cook at 400° for 10 minutes. Flip over and cook another 10 minutes*.
- Add your toppings and cook for a few minutes, or store in the fridge and use within a few days!

Recipe Notes

If you prefer a flatbread texture that is not as crispy, don't squeeze out all the water. This way you will also get about twice as many crusts.

You may want to decrease the cooking time of the crust depending upon what toppings you are putting on it. My toppings didn't need much cooking time, so after the 20 minutes of cooking the crust, I only needed to cook my pizza for a few minutes to warm it up.

Nutrition Facts
Calories 340 Calories from Fat 216
Total Fat 24g 37%
Saturated Fat 2g 10%
Cholesterol 0mg 0%
Sugars 3g
Protein 13g 26%

Vegan Zucchini Lasagna with Tofu Ricotta and Walnut Sauce

Prep Time 10 minutes
Cook Time 35 minutes
Total Time 45 minutes
Servings 4
Calories 356 kcal

Ingredients

Walnut Sauce

- cup walnuts finely ground
- 1 25 ounce jar marinara sauce, divided
- 1/4 cup sun-dried tomatoes chopped

Lasagna

- Tofu Ricotta the whole batch
- zucchini
- tablespoons nutritional yeast optional

Instructions

- Preheat oven to 375°.
- Mix walnuts, marinara sauce (reserve 3/4 cup for the pan), and sun-dried tomatoes.
- Slice zucchini 1/16" lenthwise on a mandoline.
- In an 8x9" pan, pour 3/4 cup marinara sauce. Next, place zucchini noodles on marinara sauce,

overlapping each slice. Spread 1/3 of tofu ricotta over zucchini noodles. Sprinkle nutritional yeast on top of tofu ricotta. Pour 1/2 of walnut sauce on top.

- Layer more zucchini noodles, then 1/3 of tofu ricotta, nutritional yeast, and rest of walnut sauce. Finish with layer of zucchini noodles, tofu ricotta, and nutritional yeast. Bake at 375° for 35 minutes.

Nutrition Facts
Calories 356 Calories from Fat 225
Total Fat 25g 38%
Saturated Fat 1g 5%
Cholesterol 0mg 0%
Sugars 5g

Baked Tofu Fries

Prep Time 30 minutes
Cook Time 40 minutes
Total Time 1 hour 10 minutes
Servings people
Calories 132 kcal

Ingredients

- 15.5 ounces extra firm tofu drained and pressed
- 2 tablespoons olive oil
- 1/2 teaspoon basil
- 1/2 teaspoon oregano
- 1/4 teaspoon paprika
- 1/4 teaspoon cayenne pepper
- 1/4 teaspoon onion powder
- 1/4 teaspoon garlic powder
- Salt and pepper

Instructions

- Preheat oven to 375°.
- Mix olive oil and all the herbs and spices.
- Slice tofu into long strips, about 1/4 - 1/2" thick. Coat with marinade.
- Place strips on a parchment paper lined baking sheet, and bake at 375° for 20 minutes. Flip, and bake another 15-20 minutes, or until crispy on the outside.

Nutrition Facts

Baked Tofu Fries

Calories 132 Calories from Fat 90

Total Fat 10g 15%

Saturated Fat 1g 5%

Cholesterol 0mg 0%

Hemp Seed Cauliflower Rice Pilaf

Prep Time 5 minutes
Cook Time 5 minutes
Total Time 10 minutes
Calories 208 kcal

Ingredients

- 1/2 head of cauliflower (2 cups cauliflower rice)
- 1/2 cup hemp seeds
- 4 pitted dates chopped - I used Deglet*
- 1/2 teaspoon turmeric
- 1/2 teaspoon cumin
- 1/2 low sodium vegetable broth
- 1/4 cup sliced almonds
- Salt and pepper

Instructions

- If you are using a head of cauliflower, cut it into large chunks and place in the food processor. Mix until it resembles a rice consistency.
- Place cauliflower rice in a pan along with hemp seeds, chopped dates, turmeric, cumin, vegetable broth, and salt and pepper. Cook until liquid is absorbed, about 5 minutes. Add sliced almonds.

Recipe Notes

If you are on a keto diet, you may want to use less dates, or omit them altogether.

Nutrition Facts

Calories 208 Calories from Fat 126
Total Fat 14g 22%
Saturated Fat 1g 5%
Cholesterol 0mg 0%
Sodium 5mg 0%
Potassium 133mg 4%

Ginger Sesame Walnut and Hemp Seed Lettuce Wraps

Prep Time 10 minutes
Total Time 10 minutes
Servings
Calories 382 kcal

Ingredients

Sauce

- 2 tablespoons low sodium gluten free tamari
- 1 tablespoon maple syrup
- 1 teaspoon toasted sesame oil
- 2 tablespoons brown rice vinegar
- 1 tablespoon minced ginger

Filling

- 1 cup chopped walnuts
- 1/2 cup hemp seeds
- 2 dates chopped
- 1/2 cup chopped cucumber
- 1/4 cup chopped carrots
- lettuce leaves
- sesame seeds optional

Instructions

- Mix sauce ingredients.
- Add chopped walnuts, hemp seeds, dates, cucumber, and carrots. Let sit in the fridge for at least an hour for the ingredients to combine.
- Pile mixture into lettuce leaves. Top with sesame seeds, if desired.

Nutrition Facts
Calories 382 Calories from Fat 279
Total Fat 31g 48%
Saturated Fat 2g 10%
Cholesterol 0mg 0%
Sodium 510mg 21%
Potassium 230mg 7%
Total Carbohydrates 13g

Sriracha Deviled Avocados

Prep Time 5 minutes
Total Time 5 minutes
Servings small avocados (or 2 large)
Calories 399 kcal

Ingredients

- 4 small avocados, halved and pitted (or 2 large)

Sriracha Filling

- 2 tablespoons vegan mayo
- 1/2 cup + 2 tablespoons avocado
- 4 teaspoons lime juice
- 2 tablespoons sriracha or more if you it really spicy
- 2 pinches chili powder
- salt and pepper
- paprika and cilantro for garnish

Instructions

- Mash all sriracha filling ingredients together until smooth.

- Fill the halved and pitted avocados with the deviled sriracha mixture and sprinkle paprika and cilantro on top.

Nutrition Facts
Calories 399 Calories from Fat 324
Total Fat 36g 55%
Saturated Fat 5g 25%
Cholesterol 0mg 0%
Sodium 235mg 10%
Potassium 1084mg 31%

Vegan Mashed Cauliflower with Caramelized Onions and Mushrooms

Prep Time 5 minutes
Cook Time 35 minutes
Total Time 40 minutes
Calories 56 kcal

Ingredients

- 1 head cauliflower chopped (2 cups)
- 1 tablespoon olive oil or Earth Balance
- 6 tablespoons unsweetened plain almond milk
- 1 onion chopped (2 cups)
- Salt and pepper
- Slash balsamic vinegar
- 1 cup sliced baby portobello mushrooms

Instructions

- Steam cauliflower. Set aside until cool. Mix in food processor with almond milk, salt, pepper, and olive oil or Earth Balance.
- Heat olive oil in a pan at medium low heat and add chopped onion. Stir the onion until it is coated with oil. Sprinkle a pinch of salt on the onions.
- Stir the onions every few minutes or so. Cooking will take about 20 minutes. Add balsamic vinegar to deglaze the pan after 15 minutes. Add sliced mushroom, and cook a few minutes more.

- Reheat mashed cauliflower on stovetop or in a microwave. Top with caramelized onions and mushrooms.

Nutrition Facts
Calories 56 Calories from Fat 27
Total Fat 3g 5%
Saturated Fat 0g 0%
Cholesterol 0mg 0%
Sodium 40mg 2%
Potassium 198mg 6%
Total Carbohydrates 4g

Mexican Cauliflower Rice

Prep Time 5 minutes
Cook Time 10 minutes
Total Time 15 minutes
Calories 28 kcal

Ingredients

- head of cauliflower approx. 8 cups, cut into large pieces
- 1 tablespoon olive oil
- 1/2 cup chopped onion
- cloves garlic minced
- tablespoons finely chopped serrano pepper
- 2 tablespoons tomato paste
- salt and pepper
- cilantro chopped
- limes

Instructions

- Put 1/2 the cauliflower in food processor and pulse until it resembles a rice consistency. Do the same with the other half.
- Warm olive oil in a large skillet over medium heat. Add chopped onion. Cook on medium heat until translucent.
- Add garlic and serrano pepper. Cook another minute longer.

- Add cauliflower, tomato paste, salt, and pepper. Cook until tender.
- Serve with chopped cilantro and limes.

Nutrition Facts

Calories 28 Calories from Fat 9
Total Fat 1g 2%
Saturated Fat 0g 0%
Cholesterol 0mg 0%
Sodium 36mg 2%
Potassium 106mg 3%

Tamari Seaweed Flax Crackers

Prep Time 5 minutes
dehydrate 1 day 4 hours
Total Time 5 minutes
Calories 30 kcal

Ingredients

- 1/2 cup flax seeds
- 1/2 cup golden flax seeds
- 1 1/2 cups water
- 2 tablespoon low sodium gluten free tamari
- 2 nori sheets broken up (1/2 cup)

Instructions

- Soak flaxseeds and tamari in water for at least an hour. Next, add nori. Mix thoroughly.
- Spoon 1 heaping tablespoonful per cracker on a Teflon sheet. Put in dehydrator and dehydrate at 110° for 24-28 hours, or until crispy. Turn over halfway through the dehydrating process so that they dehydrate faster.

Nutrition Facts

Calories 30 Calories from Fat 18
Total Fat 2g 3%
Saturated Fat 0g 0%
Cholesterol 0mg 0%
Sodium 69mg 3%
Potassium 48mg 1%
Total Carbohydrates 1g 0%

Sriracha Deviled Avocados

Prep Time 5 minutes
Total Time 5 minutes
Servings small avocados (or 2 large)
Calories 399 kcal

Ingredients

- 4 small avocados, halved and pitted (or 2 large)

Sriracha Filling

- 2 tablespoons vegan mayo
- 1/2 cup + 2 tablespoons avocado
- 4 teaspoons lime juice
- 2 tablespoons sriracha or more if you it really spicy
- 2 pinches chili powder
- salt and pepper
- paprika and cilantro for garnish

Instructions

- Mash all sriracha filling ingredients together until smooth.

- Fill the halved and pitted avocados with the deviled sriracha mixture and sprinkle paprika and cilantro on top.

Nutrition Facts

Calories 399 Calories from Fat 324
Total Fat 36g 55%
Saturated Fat 5g 25%
Cholesterol 0mg 0%
Sodium 235mg 10%

Vegan Pizza Football Cheese Ball

This Vegan Pizza Football Cheese Ball will be the hit of your Super Bowl party! It is easy to make, and sure to impress!

Prep Time 10 minutes
Total Time 10 minutes
Calories 94 kcal

Ingredients

- 1 (8 ounce) vegan cream cheese
- 1 (10 ounce) vegan mozzarella
- 1/4 cup sun-dried tomatoes
- 1/4 cup green olives
- 1 teaspoon basil
- 1 teaspoon oregano
- 1/2 teaspoon garlic powder
- 1/2 teaspoon onion powder
- 1 teaspoon red pepper flakes
- Salt and pepper
- 1/4 cup walnuts chopped (or other nuts)

Instructions

- Slice a small amount of vegan mozzarella off the block. Cut one long and four short strips of vegan cheese for the stripes on the football. Alternatively, you could make stripes using the vegan cream cheese.

- Mix all ingredients, except walnuts, in a food processor. Wrap vegan cheese ball in plastic wrap and let sit in the refrigerator for an hour.
- Form vegan cheese ball into a football shape. Coat in chopped walnuts. Add the stripes with vegan mozzarella or vegan cream cheese.

Nutrition Facts

Calories 94 Calories from Fat 63
Total Fat 7g 11%
Saturated Fat 2g 10%
Cholesterol 0mg 0%
Sodium 217mg 9%
Potassium 55mg 2%
Total Carbohydrates 5g

Chocolate Low Carb Vegan Fudge

This Chocolate Low Carb Vegan Fudge is melt in your mouth good! It only takes a few minutes to make with very few ingredients.

Prep Time 5 minutes
Total Time 5 minutes
Calories 97 kcal

Ingredients

- 1/2 cup cacao or cocoa powder
- 1/2 cup coconut oil melted
- 1/4 cup full fat coconut milk
- 1/2 teaspoon vanilla extract
- 1 teaspoon almond extract
- 2 teaspoons erythritol or 15-20 drops stevia
- pinch salt

Instructions

- If using erythritol, heat all ingredients in a double boiler or microwave until erythritol is dissolved. Mix all ingredients thoroughly.
- Fill either ice cube trays, muffin liners, or a plastic wrapped lined storage container. Refrigerate.
- Once cooled, if using the plastic wrapped lined container, pull fudge out and slice on a cutting board. Store in the fridge.

Recipe Notes

Nutrition facts are with erythritol, which contains 4 grams of carbs per teaspoon. So there's about 0.7 carbs in each piece of fudge, whereas stevia contains no carbs.

Nutrition Facts

Amount Per Serving
Calories 97 Calories from Fat 90
Total Fat 10g 15%
Saturated Fat 9g 45%
Cholesterol 0mg 0%
Sodium 1mg 0%
Potassium 64mg

Low Carb Vegan Almond Cookies

These healthy Low Carb Vegan Almond Cookies are a delicious low carb treat that you don't have to feel guilty about!

Prep Time 5 minutes
Cook Time 25 minutes
Total Time 30 minutes
Calories 87 kcal

Ingredients

- 1 cup almond flour super fine or the meal/ flour - both work
- 1 tablespoon flax meal
- 4 teaspoons erythritol
- 1 teaspoon baking powder
- 1/4 teaspoon salt
- 1/2 cup almond butter
- 1 teaspoon vanilla extract
- 1/2 teaspoon almond extract
- 1/2 cup unsweetened vanilla almond milk
- 4 teaspoons sliced almonds 2 per cookie

Instructions

- Preheat oven to 350°.

- Mix all dry ingredients. Add almond butter and wet ingredients.

- Mix thoroughly. Scoop tablespoonful sized balls onto a parchment paper lined baking sheet. Flatten and add two slivered almonds per cookie. Bake at 350° for 20-25 minutes or until golden.

Nutrition Facts

Calories 87 Calories from Fat 63
Total Fat 7g 11%
Saturated Fat 0g 0%
Cholesterol 0mg 0%
Sodium 42mg 2%
Potassium 83mg 2%
Total Carbohydrates 3g

Chocolate Coconut Almond Chia Pudding

This sweet Chocolate Coconut Almond Chia Pudding is made with rich coconut milk and layered with chocolate coconut almond butter.

Prep Time 5 minutes
Total Time 5 minutes
Calories 561 kcal

Ingredients

- 1/4 cup chia seeds
- 1 cup full fat coconut milk or unsweetened almond milk or a combination of the two
- 2 tablespoons cacao powder
- 1/2 teaspoon almond extract
- 1 teaspoon vanilla extract
- 1 tablespoon maple syrup or 10 drops stevia
- 2-3 tablespoons Chocolate Coconut Almond Butter*
- 2-3 tablespoons slivered almonds
- 2-3 tablespoons finely shredded coconut

Instructions

- Add coconut milk or almond milk to chia seeds. Let sit in the fridge for at least an hour.
- Add cacao powder, almond extract, vanilla extract, and maple syrup or stevia. Blend in a

Nutribullet or food processor until smooth and creamy.

- Layer pudding with Chocolate Coconut Almond Butter, slivered almonds, and coconut flakes in dessert goblets or bowls.

Recipe Notes

For a vegan keto version omit the chocolate coconut almond butter, use very little, or replace the maple syrup with stevia in that recipe.

Nutrition Facts

Calories 561 Calories from Fat 432
Total Fat 48g 74%
Saturated Fat 26g 130%
Cholesterol 0mg 0%
Sodium 23mg

Neapolitan Chia Pudding

This healthy Neapolitan Chia Pudding can be eaten for breakfast or dessert. It is easy to make and great for on the go!

Prep Time 10 minutes
Total Time 10 minutes
Servings (8) ounce jars
Calories 277 kcal

Ingredients

Chocolate layer

- 2 tablespoons chia seeds
- 1/2 cup unsweetened chocolate or vanilla almond milk
- 2 teaspoons cacao or cocoa powder
- 1/2 teaspoon vanilla extract
- 1/4 teaspoon almond extract
- 8 drops stevia

Vanilla layer

- 2 tablespoons chia seeds
- 1/2 cup unsweetened vanilla almond milk
- 1/2 teaspoon vanilla extract
- 8 drops stevia

Strawberry layer

- 1/2 cup Strawberry Chia Jam
- 6 chopped strawberries
- 4 teaspoons cacao nibs

Instructions

- Chocolate layer: Mix chia seeds and almond milk. Let sit in the fridge for at least an hour. Mix in cacao powder, vanilla extract, almond extract, and stevia.

- Vanilla layer: Mix chia seeds and almond milk. Let sit in the fridge for at least an hour. Mix in vanilla extract and stevia.

- To assemble: Divide puddings between two 8 ounce mason jars. Layer into each 1/2 of the chocolate chia pudding, then 1/2 of the vanilla chia pudding. On top of the vanilla chia pudding layer 4 tablespoons Strawberry Chia Jam. Garnish with chopped strawberries and cacao nibs.

Nutrition Facts

Calories 277 Calories from Fat 108
Total Fat 12g 18%
Saturated Fat 2g 10%
Cholesterol 0mg 0%
Sodium 167mg 7%
Potassium 308mg

Pumpkin Chia Pudding

This smooth and creamy Pumpkin Chia Pudding is not only easy to make, but is healthy enough to be eaten for breakfast.

Prep Time 1 hour 5 minutes
Total Time 1 hour 5 minutes
Calories 138 kcal

Ingredients

- 1/4 cup chia seeds
- cup unsweetened vanilla almond milk
- 1 teaspoon vanilla extract
- 15-20 drops stevia or 2 dates softened in hot water
- 1/4 cup pumpkin puree
- 1/2 teaspoon pumpkin spice
- pinch salt
- chopped pecans

Instructions

- Mix chia seeds and almond milk. Let sit in the fridge for at least an hour.
- Add vanilla extract, stevia or dates, pumpkin puree, pumpkin spice, and salt.
- Mix in a high speed blender or Nutribullet until smooth and creamy. Garnish with chopped pecans.

Nutrition Facts

Calories 138 Calories from Fat 72
Total Fat 8g 12%
Saturated Fat 0g 0%
Cholesterol 0mg 0%
Sodium 167mg 7%
Potassium 149mg 4%
Total Carbohydrates

Keto Chicken Pot Pie

Cook Time22 mins
Course: Main Course
Servings: 8 servings
Calories: 297kcal

Ingredients

For the Chicken Pot Pie Filling:

- 2 tablespoons of butter
- 1/2 cup mixed veggies could also substitute green beans or broccoli
- 1/4 small onion diced
- 1/4 tsp pink salt
- 1/4 tsp pepper
- 2 garlic cloves minced
- 3/4 cup heavy whipping cream
- 1 cup chicken broth
- 1 tsp poultry seasoning
- 1/4 tsp rosemary
- pinch thyme
- 2 1/2 cups cooked chicken diced
- 1/4 tsp Xanthan Gum

For the crust:

- 4 1/2 tablespoons of butter melted and cooled
- 1/3 cup coconut flour

- 2 tablespoons full fat sour cream
- 4 eggs
- 1/4 teaspoon salt
- 1/4 teaspoon baking powder
- 1 1/3 cup sharp shredded cheddar cheese or mozzarella shredded

Instructions

- Cook 1 to 1 1/2 lbs chicken in the slow cooker for 3 hours on high or 6 hours on low.
- Preheat oven to 400 degrees.
- Sautee onion, mixed veggies, garlic cloves, salt, and pepper in 2 tablespoons butter in an oven safe skillet for approx 5 min or until onions are translucent.
- Add heavy whipping cream, chicken broth, poultry seasoning, thyme, and rosemary.
- Sprinkle Xanthan Gum on top and simmer for 5 minutes so that the sauce thickens. Make sure to simmer covered as the liquid will evaporate otherwise. You need a lot of liquid for this recipe, otherwise, it will be dry.
- Add diced chicken.
- Make the breading by combining melted butter (I cool mine by popping the bowl in the fridge for 5 min), eggs, salt, and sour cream in a bowl then whisk together.
- Add coconut flour and baking powder to the mixture and stir until combined.
- Stir in cheese.

- Drop batter by dollops on top of the chicken pot pie. Do not spread it out, as the coconut flour will absorb too much of the liquid.
- Bake in a 400-degree oven for 15-20 min.
- Set oven to broil and move chicken pot pie to top shelf. Broil for 1-2 minutes until bread topping is nicely browned.

Nutrition

Calories: 297kcal | Carbohydrates: 5.3g | Protein: 11.6g | Fat: 17g | Fiber: 2g

Easy Stir Fry Kimchi & Pork Belly

Stir-fry kimchi and bork belly is so simple to make yet out of this world satisfying! Dinner under 30 minutes, and Keto friendly.

Prep Time5 mins
Cook Time: 15 mins
Marinating: Time10 mins
Total Time: 20 mins
Servings: 3 people
Calories: 804 kcal

Ingredients

- 300 g naturally-raised pork belly
- 1 tbsp naturally-brewed tamari or soy sauce (gluten-free option: use tamari or gluten-free soy sauce)
- 1 tbsp naturally-brewed rice wine
- 1 lb kimchi (see notes below)
- 1 stalk green onion
- 1 tbsp sesame seeds (optional)

Instructions

- Slice the pork belly as thin as possible. Marinate in tamari/soy sauce and rice wine for about 10 minutes. If your kimchi isn't pre-cut, then cut into 1 inch size.

- Heat a heavy bottom pan (I use cast iron). While the pan is very hot, add the marinated pork belly, stir fry until nicely browned, for approximately 5 to 10 minutes. You should see some fat being cooked out of the pork belly at this point.

- Add the kimchi into the pan, stir-fry for another 2 minutes, for the flavour of kimchi and pork to completely mix.

- Turn off the heat. Thinly slice the green onion, and add to the stir fry.

- If available, sprinkle sesame seeds on top as garnish.

Recipe Notes

If you use a store-bought kimchi, make sure to check the ingredients. I use a home-made fermented kimchi that's free of MSG and added sugar.

CONCLUSION

The keto plan is a versatile and interesting way to lose weight, with lots of delicious food choices.

To thrive on the vegan diet, it is important to cover any nutrient deficiencies you may have from exclusively eating plant foods.